The information included in this book is for educational purposes only. It is not intended or implied to be a substitute for professional medical advice. The reader should always consult his or her healthcare provider to determine the appropriateness of the information for his or her own situation or if he or she has any questions concerning a medical condition or treatment plan.

Dedications

There are so many people I could thank who have contributed willingly and also unknowingly to make this book possible. Firstly, my parents Doris and Harold, who created me and laid the foundation for my life in my youth. Then all of my work colleagues and employees who believed in my vision in business which created success and allowed me to travel the world and develop a broad understanding of what life is all about and how to appreciate this planet we call home.

My children, who have always been part of me and who created my grandchildren which produced that "stop and think" moment that changed the course of my life. It made me more aware of my own mortality and encouraged me to search out ways where I could remain on this Earth as long as possible.

I must thank the Cornerstone Christian Church in Chandler, Arizona. They provided me with the platform to guide me from being a non-believer to a Christian, which changed me on the inside. It has allowed me to deal with personal struggles and also forced me to deal with my own mortality.

My special thanks to all those scientists and researchers who spend their lives trying to find solutions to our health problems. Their incessant search for answers leads us to the possibilities we are discussing in this book. This has also led to the successful replacement of my aortic valve - twice! Without these developments I would never have come this far.

Last but not least, I have to thank my wife Ingrid. She too was forced to make the journey from "traditional" nutrition to something different which was not so easy for her. Her pleasure and special skill has always been preparing fantastic meals for me every single day. Suddenly, we were skipping meals and mixing smoothies, a world that was new for her. Vielen Dank Liebling!

Preface

Intermittent Fasting is becoming one of the latest rages in the dieting community and has been often dubbed as a fad solution to weight-loss. This is very unfortunate as this cannot be farther from the truth. There are several books you can buy on **Intermittent Fasting** and most of them appear between other books on various dieting and weight-loss programs. Therefore, I have written this book to try and change the focus on this revolutionary, lifestyle-changing phenomenon called fasting.

One of our desires as individuals is to live a **happy, healthy and longer life**. Sometimes we forget this goal and succumb to the so-called excesses and pleasures of modern society. Then we rely upon the fact that, on-average, life expectancy has been on the increase for decades anyway and "by the time we get there" it will have increased even more. This is a dangerous assumption.

We live on a planet which is divided into two completely separate segments of population - developed and underdeveloped nations, or as some people would characterize them as rich and poor. It has been popular belief (also for me) that in the developed nations of the world life expectancy is longer than in the poorer nations because we have better access to healthcare which keeps us alive longer. This is partly true but is not the main reason for the increase in life expectancy.

The term life expectancy typically refers to how long we can expect to live at the moment of birth. In the USA this figure on average for men is 76 years and for women 81. It has been increasing steadily over the past decades but has now flattened out and in the USA it has actually started to decline. One of the biggest impacts on this average number is not access to healthcare but the elimination of death at birth, which has been almost eradicated in richer countries and drastically reduced in the underdeveloped world. By eliminating the number of deaths at birth, the average life expectancy statistic increases quickly but as this impact becomes less of a factor, the life expectancy increase starts to slow or even fall, as is now the case in some countries.

What we also forget is our life expectancy increases as we get older. in the USA a man reaching the age of 60 can now expect to live until 81 and a woman 84. I am now 73 and my average life expectancy has risen to 85!

Why is all this so important? What has been happening in western societies is the average life expectancy has been on the increase for the reasons mentioned above, but so has the number of deaths from the diseases of modern society. An example I cover extensively in this book is being overweight and obesity. This has been on a steady increase over the past decades and has proven to be the cause of many of the diseases we die from with more than 70% of the population in the USA falling into this category.

As the increase in life expectancy slows and starts to decrease because of these diseases, ways to avoid and even eliminate them, not just treating them, becomes an ever important factor. Of course, if you like playing the lottery then this might not be a problem but if you feel you would like to increase your odds of a longer, healthier life then I have an answer for you. It is called **Intermittent Fasting**.

In fact, I believe we are on the cusp of a real revolution when it comes to staying healthy and living longer which will have a huge impact on our society as a whole. Just imagine what would happen if we could eliminate or drastically reduce obesity, diabetes, cardio vascular diseases, stroke, cancer, dementia, Alzheimer's, Parkinson's disease and many more. Not only would we increase the average life expectancy, we would revolutionize the healthcare industry. This may sound like a very pretentious claim but I hope after you have read this book you will understand the power of what I am proposing and join the many thousands who have already embarked on this journey.

My sales pitch is this is a book for beginners and is therefore named "The Beginner's Guide". It lays out in simple terms what **Intermittent Fasting** is all about, background information in non-medical language and proposes a simple plan to get started. You will lose weight and burn fat with **Intermittent Fasting** but you will also achieve much, much more. The good news is it is simple, will cost you nothing and is safe. You can try it and if it is not for you you can stop! **A Trial Of One**.

TABLE OF CONTENTS

The Author

My name is Colin Buckingham, I am a Brit, 73 years old, a father of three and a grandad of four. I am not a doctor, nor a scientist, nor a sports trainer, nor a physician, nor a dietitian, nor a naturopath. So why am I sitting here writing about something that can change your health so dramatically it could knock at least ten years or more off your biological clock, help you avoid many of the diseases which could kill you and help you live a healthier, longer life? What could be my motivation? The answer to this question is simple and a combination of different things.

First of all and, most importantly, I have personally gone though what I am proposing here and can talk from real life experience. When I compare where my body was before I started my plan and where it was after just 90 days, I can honestly say that my health, which includes everything from my weight to my blood markers and how I feel, improved so much I estimate it turned my biological clock back more than ten years. I want you to achieve the same success. I am not a so-called fitness expert trying to sell you the latest dieting fad. In fact my plan will cost you nothing and you could even save money on groceries.

Therefore, I can claim to be an **"Expert of Experts"** as I have read almost every book on **Intermittent Fasting** and studied hundreds of scientific experiments on the subject and watched dozens of informational videos before I tried it. For the past ten years I have also been following the new science called **Nutrigenomics** and have listened to scores of presentations on how researchers are discovering new ways to influence our genetic makeup with things we ingest. I have been able to analyze this information and formulate conclusions which are not influenced by any profit motives and I have implemented these into my own life. I want others to have the chance to benefit from the same knowledge.

Another big motivation for me to take the time to put pen to paper is I love writing. Back in my grammar school days in the UK, I used to win every English essay competition they came up with. People also comment on my ability to see the big picture. The ability to focus on the causes of poor health and not the symptoms. Many have suggested that I outsource the actual writing of this book to an agency (which many authors do) but for me the fun has been in the journey not just the destination.

To round off my bio, I consider myself a global citizen, have lived in six different countries, speak five languages fluently, have traveled the world extensively, successfully managed large corporations, built and sold my own business, hosted kings and princes, have run three half-marathons in my retirement and recently biked from Berlin to Stuttgart (900 km) in ten days.

None of this might be relevant to the subject matter of this book but could indicate how broad my insight is on a wide range of subjects concerning health and attitude to life on this planet. It is a beautiful place and we should do our utmost to spend as much time as we can enjoying its riches and its diversity.

I believe we are on the brink of some major changes in the healthcare industry and the time has come for **all of us** to take control of our own health and destiny. **Intermittent Fasting** offers us the opportunity to implement a plan which will allow us to live a healthier and longer life and change the way we view nutrition and how the food and healthcare industries sell us their products and services. A revolution.

These are massive forces which will do their utmost to stop this revolution as their huge profits and wealth are at risk. I just hope you will absorb this information, implement some (or all) of the suggestions, experience the benefits that will come and then pass on this information to your family and friends. This is the only way we can create a revolution and experience better health and the chance of a longer life.

1. INTRODUCTION

The Beginner's Guide

When I decided to sit down and write, I had just one aim in mind - to try and convince as many people as I can to try **Intermittent Fasting**. It's pretty clear. **Intermittent Fasting** is simple to implement, will cost you nothing and has an almost unlimited number of benefits which could help you live a healthier and potentially longer life. I spent months of in-depth research on the subject of fasting before I decided to give it a try. It has worked and is working for me.

I am now conveying this knowledge in a form which should be easy to understand so you can also be convinced to give it a try. I have collected some of the documents I have read and the videos I have watched in the Appendices section so you don't have to spend time searching for this information. I lay out a simple **Intermittent Fasting Plan** which is easy to understand and implement. Try it and if it doesn't work for you then stop! You have everything to gain and nothing to lose.

Once I wrote a magazine article entitled **"The Expert Of Experts"** which points out that most experts are almost never completely right. This is particularly true on the subjects of health, aging and disease. If you ask the question, "What is the cause of aging?" you will get at least ten different answers, all backed up by scientific research! "What is the best method to burn body fat?". At last five different methods. So it often takes people like me, with **no financial benefit** from any one particular solution, to sort through the noise and come up with a balanced conclusion and suggestions. An expert of experts.

The subject in this book is the new but ancient philosophy of fasting, how it works and how you can benefit from it to live a healthier and disease-free life. Many of the publications about fasting have either been written by scientists, researchers or so-called experts in a form normal folks like you and I cannot understand or it is so superficial it doesn't really cover the subject matter extensively enough. Oftentimes it is a ploy from a so-called expert to sell you something. This is not the case here. The actual **Intermittent Fasting Plan** is relatively straightforward and easy to follow which is why I will spend more time on background information and arguments which will help motivate you to move forward.

After doing three months of solid research before my first fast, I discovered that fasting has never been a mainstream, recommended method of **improving health**, **extending life**, and **avoiding** and maybe even **curing** many of the diseases that kill us. Even my own doctor admitted he had "heard something about fasting" but actually he knew nothing about it! So I thought it was time to get the word out. I will be spending more time on covering the health aspects of fasting than just the pure weight-loss benefit and my goal is to describe this phenomenon in a form that the average person can understand. A Beginner's Guide.

Background

This is not the first book about **Intermittent Fasting**. In fact, I have read almost all of the others. They are either too scientific, not easy for the average person to comprehend or they are too superficial and sometimes badly structured. In almost all cases they were often written with the intention of taking the reader down a certain path which leads to buying another product or service. This is not the case here. I outline the fasting plan in detail which you can follow without having to spend another cent. In fact, as you will learn, you will actually save some money by eating less.

You will discover by just skipping one meal daily you can lose those unwanted pounds of fat, clean out the abuse you may have committed to your body in the past and avoid most of the deadly diseases that could kill you and therefore live a much healthier, longer life. How can I make such a claim? The answer is overwhelming scientific proof, common-sense and my own personal experience.

Let me just mention a couple of things you might be doing already and accept as normal. If you suffer from a headache, you might take an aspirin or another pain killer. My question is **why**? Did you study all the FDA testing on how the chemical components of the pain killers react with your nerve cells and numb the pain? Or did you take it because it works? If your headache had been caused by a more serious, underlying illness, did the pain killer actually cure that illness?

The sale of pain killers is an annual, **multi-billion dollar business** but do you believe they actually resolve the cause of the headache? No, they just relieve the symptoms. In fact many of the medicines in the multi-trillion dollar drug business only relieve symptoms and don't cure the illness. If pharmaceutical companies were to develop real cures it would put them out of business!

A good example is diabetes which has become one of the biggest killers in western society. It can cause a long list of related diseases including heart attacks, stroke, cancer, Alzheimer's, Parkinson's and many more. Hundreds of millions of people inject insulin into their bodies every single day, sometimes more than once. Does this cure diabetes? No. In fact, science has now proven that these injections force people to gain more weight and which makes the disease even worse. The real problem is this almost guarantees a shorter life with the risk of developing one or more of some debilitating disease.

If you had diabetes and one of the world's leading experts on diabetes is proposing that by following an **Intermittent Fasting Program**, diabetes could not only be cured, it could be prevented from even happening in the first place, would you be interested? What if he had patients who had achieved this result by following his advice, would you even consider it as being possible? Well, this person exists and his name is Dr. Jason Fung from Toronto, Canada and I have included links to a number of presentations about his findings and philosophy at the end of the book under Appendix D.

It is unlikely you will get such advice from experts being financed by the pharmaceutical companies about how to deal with many of the diseases that keep them in business and which could potentially kill you. Recent scientific discoveries have now emerged about a wide range of health benefits of a simple **Intermittent Fasting** regime. These benefits have been scientifically proven to help avoid many of the killer diseases we die from and, in some cases, even cure ailments like diabetes. This is information you will not be getting from the established industries which profit from your bad health.

This threat to business interests which **Intermittent Fasting** poses has led to many misconceptions being published on the subject of fasting. Here are just a few you might have already seen or could come across:

- You will enter a starvation mode and always be hungry

- Fasting will break down your muscle mass

- You will become undernourished

- Your metabolism will decrease

- Your blood sugar levels will become too low

- Once you start eating normally again, you will regain the weight and more

- Breakfast is the most important meal of the day (so don't miss it!)

- Starving yourself is just plain unhealthy

- The testing has only been carried out on animals

None of these statements are true and cannot be verified by any type of research or from any practical case studies but are thrown around by those industries and individuals with business interests which are threatened by the implementation of a fasting regime. This leads to contradictory opinions and sometimes dangerous assumptions and statements being made which are not always in your best interest. A later chapter deals with this issue in more detail so it will suffice here to point out that the food processing and packaging industry, the healthcare industry, the food supplements industry and the dieting industry all have profits at risk if everyone started to fast and became healthy.

So, if you are open to looking at a few simple adjustments to how you live your life, which will cost you nothing and give you added energy and mental focus, then this is the moment to read on! Clear your mind of all your preconceived notions of health, diet, losing weight and exercise and adopt something that is working for a growing number of people around the world. **Intermittent Fasting**. Healthier and more effective than taking an Aspirin. Try it and you will see it works!

Your Body

Your body is probably one of the most valued possessions you have. Without it you would be nobody. But you have it and one of the questions you should be asking is, are you taking good care of it? There is a lot at stake. Whether it be just for your own health, wellbeing and lifespan but also for others who depend upon you. This could include your children, your parents, your grandchildren, your loved ones, maybe your co-workers or even employees. Everyone who might depend on you and is planning on you being around for a while. However, to keep things simple **let's just focus on you**.

Your body is one of the marvels of our universe. With the rapid advances in science and technology we are beginning only recently to understand how this intricate machine we call the human body functions and how all of its component parts work together to give you a life worth living. Remaining healthy and living a long life has occupied humans for centuries, driven by the fear of disease and death. It is not a stretch of the imagination to understand that taking good care of your body is just like taking good care of your automobile.

With your car you feed it with gasoline, make sure the tire and oil pressures are maintained, you wash it occasionally and then send it to the workshop for a maintenance checkup every so often. You may have much of the same routine for your body. But there is just one problem. Your body is much more complex than your automobile and there are a thousand and one more things that can go wrong leading to disease and death.

Therefore, you should be paying **much more attention** to your body than your auto. This is something not many of us do. Life gets in the way. There are so many other distractions we have to deal with every day, whether it be getting the kids to school, getting to work on time, doing the shopping, cleaning the house or apartment, managing schedules, dealing with conflicts and so on and so on. In the midst of all these life events, how often do you sit down and ponder how your body is dealing with all of this?

When we are young, much of this is not a problem. Our bodies are healthy and are able to deal with the stress we put it through. Unfortunately, under the surface problems could be brewing which don't surface until later in life. These can include many of the diseases that kill us. Cardiovascular problems, diabetes, cancer and finally dementia and Alzheimer's. These are all silent diseases that don't just develop overnight but are often caused by the lack of thought and attention we give our body during the course of our life. The good news is, in many cases, they can be avoided if we just pay a little more attention to our body **EVERY DAY**.

Are there any symptoms we could recognize that might be warning signs of things going wrong? Yes there are. Besides smoking cigarettes which almost guarantees you will not live a long and healthy life, there are other signs that are easily recognizable as huge risks to your health. The big one in the western economies is obesity and generally being overweight. This is a phenomenon which has only emerged during the last 100 years and can be labeled one of the "diseases of the modern era".

Being overweight invariably means our bodies carry too much fat which is stored just in case we might face the famine, which never comes. In the United States it has reached epidemic proportions. A recent study shows that 70.2% of the US population is either obese or overweight (37.7% obese, 32.5% overweight). This is established by measuring the BMI index (Body Mass Index). With a BMI of 25 to 30 one is considered overweight and above 30 obese (above 40 extreme obese). Even without calculating our BMI, most of us know if we are overweight or not. The most common symptom is our clothes start to fit tight and we have to loosen our belts a notch or two!

The costs of being obese or overweight to any nation are enormous. In the USA alone one estimates that it costs the government around **$200 billion** in **extra** healthcare costs **every year**. It is one of the major causes behind such diseases as cancer, diabetes, cardiovascular problems, Alzheimer's and Parkinson's, just to mention a few. It also has a major impact on industrial productivity as obesity creates a much higher absenteeism rate in industry with costs running into billions of dollars. The other problem is that obesity is on the increase. In the USA, obesity in adults has doubled since the 1980's and tripled in children.

In the United Kingdom (UK), the picture is similar. A study by the WHO (World Health Organization) in 2014 rated the obese as 28.1% of the adult population and 33.9% as overweight. Of the children, 17% were obese and 14% overweight. The bigger problem in the UK is obesity is on the rise at a much faster rate and has quadrupled in just the last 25 years.

So this is one of the obvious signs we can all see that things are going in the wrong direction. It is a sign we are allowing our environment to get the better of us and we are not paying attention to how we treat our bodies and our overall health.

Overweight And Obesity

Being overweight invariably means our bodies carry too much fat. Fat that is stored just in case we have to face the famine, which never comes. In the United States it has reached epidemic proportions. As mentioned before, a recent study shows that 70.2% of the US population is either obese or overweight (37.7% obese, 32.5% overweight).

These types of statistics beg the question: Why is this happening and what can be done about it? For starters it is the food industry supplying us with an endless supply of processed foods which come out of factories loaded with sugars and chemicals. It is also our own fault for not taking care of ourselves and sometimes pure ignorance of what we are doing to our own bodies. But then again, its not quite as simple as that.

Obesity is not only caused by what we eat and when we eat it. There are some other components we should be aware of. The big one is the ever declining amount of physical exercise we expose our bodies to. It doesn't take much to understand today's generation exerts its body to much less physical activity than a few decades ago.

We sit around all day - at least the majority of us do. We drive to work, we drive to the supermarket, we drive our kids to school. We even try and pick the parking spot closest to the front door of the supermarket or shopping center so we don't have to walk too far. Our most strenuous sport might be trying to beat our kids playing tennis on the Playstation! We watch TV, drive to the movies, take the elevator not the stairs and then wonder why we gain weight.

Eating the wrong things is one of the problems but equally our resistance to any form of physical exercise is the other. Here is a list of the many recognized benefits you can enjoy with regular exercise:

- reduce your risk of a heart attack

- manage your weight better

- lower your blood cholesterol level

- lower the risk of type 2 diabetes and some cancers

- have lower blood pressure

- stronger bones, muscles and joints and lower the risk of osteoporosis

- lower your risk of falling

- recover better from a period of hospitalization or bed rest

- more energy, a better mood, feel more relaxed and sleep better

Any of these items sound familiar? Many of them are similar to the benefits which can be achieved through **Intermittent Fasting**. This is not surprising as physical exercise also promotes the burning of sugar and then excess fat in the body. Firstly, it helps burn the glucose in the bloodstream and accelerates the time it takes to get the body into a state of ketosis (fat burning). This is why regular exercise enhances greatly the fasting experience.

What do we mean with "physical exercise"? A health club membership? Actually not. All it takes is to look for moments in your daily life when you can be physically active. Park the car further away from the shopping center entrance, take the stairs instead of the elevator, go for a walk in the evening with your partner or family, try and do the shopping by bike instead of the car. In my family we hardly ever use the automobile in the summer! Most websites proposing physical activity will advise you to plan walking 30 minutes three or four days each week. That's all.

Of course, investing in a set of dumbbells at home is not forbidden nor is a treadmill or static bike but try the other things first and try and do them with your family and/or friends. Not only is it good for your health, maybe it will contribute to your relationships as well.

2. INTERMITTENT FASTING

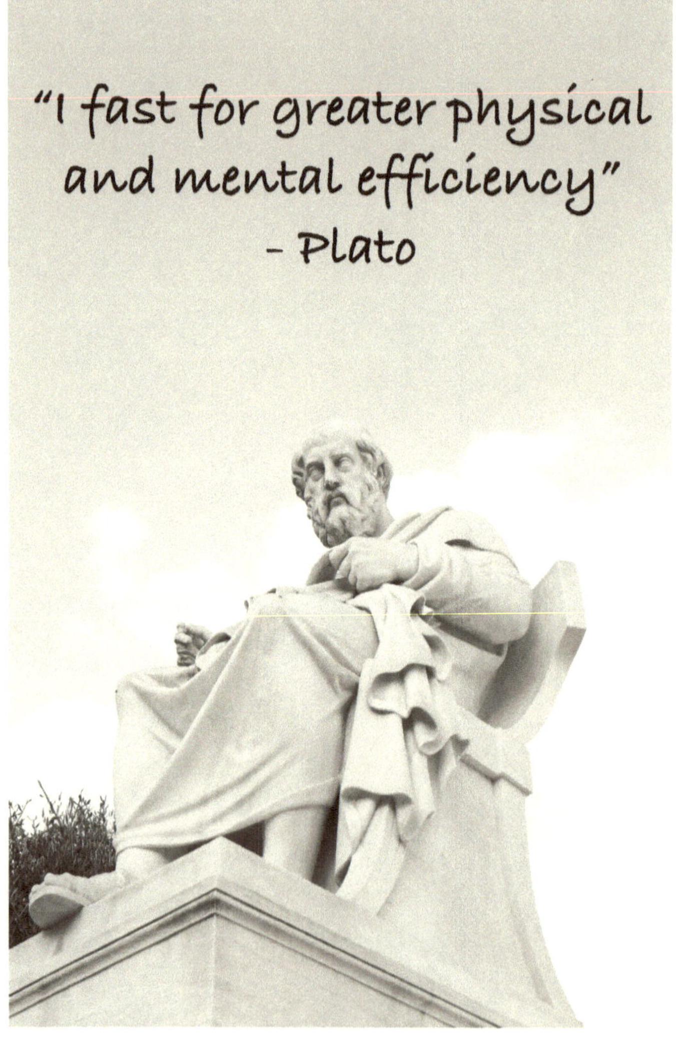

What Is Intermittent Fasting?

First of all, fasting is one of the oldest eating plans known to man. It has been practiced by humans since the time we became human beings. In the days of the caveman, the male was responsible for nourishing his family and his female partner took care of the cave and the children. In other words the male was the hunter.

Did the family eat three meals every day? Was breakfast their most important meal of the day? No. They ate after every successful hunting expedition. This meant they often went days without food and in colder climates these periods without food were often much longer. Some scientists claim that this natural start/stop eating process has been long since programmed into our genes and is therefore something we can adapt to naturally today.

Fasting has also been practiced by almost all the religions of the world for centuries. It is seen as a way to clear the mind of the burdens of the past and the present to enable a refocus on the future. A type of reset button. It is seen as a method to rid the body of the indulgences of daily life to enable a free, spiritual state of mind, and the ability to see things in a different perspective.

Here are a few quotes from famous philosophers from the past who have fasted:

"I fast for greater physical and mental efficiency" - Plato

"Fasting is the greatest remedy - the physician within" - Paracelsus

"The best of all medicines is resting and fasting" - Benjamin Franklin

"Humans live on one quarter of what they eat; on the other three quarters lives their doctor" - Egyptian Pyramid Inscription, 3800 B.C.

Please note that these quotes are not talking about losing weight but about living healthier! Therefore, I claim that fasting, and in my case, **Intermittent Fasting** (IF), is the oldest and best-kept health secret of all time. **Intermittent Fasting** has only really emerged in the past decade as a subject of increased interest. Philosophers in the past have experienced the benefits and the effects of fasting but only in the recent decade have scientists really been able to research and discover exactly what happens in the human body and to human cells when we stop eating.

These benefits were first discovered when the fasting plans lasted several days, and in some cases weeks, without food. Later it has been proven that the same benefits are attainable when shorter periods of fasting are used. Currently, **Intermittent Fasting** includes a number of plans where we restrict our food intake to certain periods of the day or week. Thus one secret behind **Intermittent Fasting** is it addresses not **WHAT** we eat but **WHEN** we eat. By giving our body a rest from the continuous process of eating and digestion, it has been discovered the body then has more time to regenerate itself.

The better known **Intermittent Fasting** plans are the so-called 16/8 and 5/2 schedules. 8 hours of eating and 16 hours of fasting every day (16/8) or 5 days of eating and 2 days of fasting every week (5/2). Another plan, which I have used in an adapted form, is the so-called Alternative Day Fast (24/24). In its simplest form one eats for a 24-hour period and then fasts for the next 24 hours. This is then repeated for the length of the plan.

In my adapted version I ate breakfast every single day (so I could take my medications). On my fasting day I didn't eat my next meal until breakfast the following day (24 hours later). This was my 24-hour fast. I then ate three normal meals the next day, my eating day, and then repeated my fasting day. More about this later.

So here is the big question: **Why should you even consider Intermittent Fasting?**

Well, maybe I can help you with this question by describing my own motivations. As I mentioned before, I have lived a pretty healthy life: never smoked, drink occasionally, exercise regularly, no drugs, eat consciously, take supplements. But I had heart problems and I was not completely happy with my weight, which had increased considerably over the past ten years. With the arrival of my grandkids, life began to take on a new meaning with new responsibilities.

Having reached the age of 73, I was becoming more aware of my own mortality and decided I just want to live as long as I possibly can. Then one day I came across a video on the Internet about fasting. It is a kind of a documentary on the subject of fasting where a BBC reporter by the name of Michael Mosley went on a journey looking for a way to live longer, stay younger and lose weight. On this quest he came across the new developments in the area of fasting.

After some very sobering base tests, he discovered he was at risk for a number of diseases, including cardiovascular problems and cancer. He was not obese but had an excess of fat, particularly around his abdomen (waist). This brought him in contact with expert researchers in the area of fasting and led him to some amazing discoveries. I strongly recommend you watch this documentary and you will find the link to this video at the end of the book. This was the start of my path of discovery and maybe it could be yours.

Michael's message was so convincing, it launched me on my own journey that changed my life. After spending the next three months researching every corner of the Internet to absorb all the information that exits on fasting, I decided to embark on the journey myself to eliminate more than 10 years from my biological clock. My attitude was it would cost me nothing to try, it is not dangerous so what do I have to lose? In my direct environment I had no supporters as nobody had tried it themselves so I was basically on my own.

Why Is Intermittent Fasting Controversial?

If you do a search on the Web about **Intermittent Fasting** you will find lots of question marks and, in some cases, a number of negative articles. Why is this the case? The main reason is that **Intermittent Fasting** far outcompetes all other concepts to lose weight and improve health. Of course, if you have been selling the idea of counting calories (Weight Watchers), following a ketogenic diet or any other type of weight-loss diet, then **Intermittent Fasting** can be a real threat.

But if we summarize what has happened over the past few decades, the population as a whole as gotten fatter and fatter which means these other solutions aren't working. When it comes to the overwhelming scientific evidence that fasting does work, you will often read "but the trials have only been carried out on animals and we will have to wait for human trials". This is nonsense as ALL medical trials are first carried out on animals, especially those of the big drug makers who are threatened by a nation which could fast its way to good health.

The great philosophers didn't wait for clinical trials as they didn't exist then. They fasted because it worked. I call this **"The trial of ONE"**! This concept is pretty simple. You try it and if it doesn't work for you, you stop it. There are hundreds of thousands, including myself, who have tried it and it has worked. I don't need to wait for some research funded by Weight Watchers or a drug company which tries to prove their system is better.

The truth of the matter is **Intermittent Fasting** has come to the forefront more recently **just because** science has now shown it has so many more health benefits than just losing weight. This I will cover at greater length in the Chapter "The Science". The

Food Processing Industry, the Medical Profession, the Pharmaceutical Industry and even the government are all powerful lobbies which would prefer **Intermittent Fasting** goes away.

Opposing Forces - The Illness Industry

We follow the advice of experts all our lives. Our parents, of course, on life in general, our teachers at school for the academics and then all the other professions such as doctors, scientists, personal trainers, dietitians, physicians and so on. The reason we do this is we assume, and probably correctly, that these individuals have been educated to higher degree in their professions than we are. They just know more about their stuff.

This may be true but there is just one small problem that infiltrates this advice. It's that small thing called "MONEY". The main reason why these well-educated individuals spend years of their lives and considerable amounts of money educating themselves is mostly so they can practice their noble professions and create an income. In my view, this is where taking advice from experts can sometimes be a problem. Their advice is often prejudiced by financial interests.

Let's take a look at a few of the above-named professionals. I will start with doctors as they often get involved with our health (or illnesses) and this will include your house doctor and any other type of specialist you might have been in contact with. When we have a problem we naturally turn to them for advice. Here is my problem.

Where is the focus of their advice and how do they get paid?

In the case of focus, it seems fairly obvious the vast majority in the medical profession only deals with you when you have a problem. You break a leg, have constant headaches, high blood pressure or something hurts somewhere, you go to the doctor. Then the wheels start to turn. Your house doctor orders all sorts of tests to try and analyze what's going on. Having gotten the results you are then passed on to a specialist who is hopefully an expert on your particular ailment(s) or disease.

My question is simply this: where are all the medical professionals who are involved in prevention, before you get sick? As you may have gathered already, one main themes of this book is to watch what and when you eat as it has a major effect on your body and your health. In the USA I have been told that of the 5 years training a medical professional puts him or herself through to practice medicine, only **20 hours**

are dedicated to nutrition! Sounds a little crazy, but true.

So the whole chain reaction from your house doctor through to specialists and the surgeons in hospitals only helps deal with the problem once it has developed. Millions of specialists, trillions of dollars. Now that this "Illness System" is in place, nobody has any financial motivation in preventing diseases and preventing the causes of the problem. I have tried to calculate exactly how many jobs are involved in this "illness" process in the USA and it is not easy to estimate. But if I include every single resource and job connected to the medical industry such as administrative functions, distribution, hospital building and management services, medical equipment manufacturers, insurance companies and of course the government, then it could be approaching 20% of the total population or more.

Do you think there might be a very powerful lobby against a national disease prevention campaign which would marginalize many of these jobs?

Let me now turn to the **pharmaceutical companies** (Big Pharma). Here is another trillion dollar industry involved in treating diseases, not curing them. In fact, they work hand-in-hand with the healthcare providers because they are their main distribution channel. This colossus of an industry only survives on illness, not good health. Do you think they are working flat out on preventive solutions to all the diseases they currently treat? That would put them out of business!

In fact the FDA (Federal Drug Administration, The Government), which is totally financed by Big Pharma, has a stranglehold on any potential groundbreaking disease-preventive solutions. That is why for every promising, natural wellness solution you will always see the following text *"These statements have not been evaluated by the Food and Drug Administration. These products are not intended to diagnose, treat, cure or prevent disease"*, even if there is anecdotal evidence to prove they do. The government also has no interest in changing anything. Big Pharma and the medical profession provides a huge, steady, tax income.

Opposing Forces - The Food Industry

Last, but definitely not least, I must talk about **the food industry** separately, which is probably the main cause of illnesses in our western democracies. If you accept the fact that being obese or overweight is one of the causes, and probably the main cause, of many of the lethal diseases, then there has to be some connection with what we are eating and these killers. Not just the quantity of food but also the quality.

If we go back to less than 75 years ago, and think carefully, what were people eating then? Initially, many families were happy if they got anything to eat at all, especially in war-ravaged Europe. People scraped together anything they could find and either grew their own vegetables or bought from the farmers directly to be able to afford anything decent.

As the decades passed, this picture changed dramatically. Local shopkeepers emerged with their individual shops selling their specialities (Butcher, Baker and Candlestick Maker). But gradually things took a different turn. Food went from a necessity to survive and developed into a lucrative, mass-producing industry. Capitalists came to realize that everyone has to eat and this is the basis of a great business model. Every day, every week, every month, potential customers have to commit a certain percentage of their incomes to food. In fact food is often the second biggest expense of anyone's budget after their living quarters.

The local high streets with their butchers, bakers and grocery stores started to disappear. In their place emerged supermarkets, where one could shop more conveniently and buy everything one needed in one place. The product supply chains to these stores also started to change. Supermarkets began to offer packaged foods in convenient containers for consumers who had no time or desire to be standing in the kitchen preparing meals. The food packaging companies came to realize they were now in a very lucrative business and competition emerged. Now they started promoting food to the consumer not based on good nutrition but on shareholder satisfaction. Big Business.

Their attention began to focus on producing their products as cheaply as possible so their profit margins satisfied the demands of their investors, not the nutrition requirements of their customers. A good example of this is the introduction of fructose as a sweetener. Fructose (HFCS) is a by-product of corn and has no connection with sugar cane but is extremely cheap to produce. Now almost all processed foods are sweetened with HFCS which is unhealthy for the consumer and it is claimed to be one of the main causes of the diabetes epidemic.

The next step in this process was the consolidation of the big supermarkets. They discovered bigger is better and even more profitable, started to merge together and found it easier to increase profits. With the larger volume, however, came the industrialization of the industry. Food providers today are large factories, highly automated and are able to execute even more price pressure on farmers and other raw material providers.

Because of this pressure farmers were forced to intensify the use of pesticides to ward off attacks from insects and to increase the return on their harvests. Scientists worked hard on gene manipulation to make crops grow faster and resist more disease. Animals no longer have the pleasure of seeing the light of day but instead are cooped up in enclosures where they cannot even move and are forced fed so they put on weight unnaturally.

At the same time, both the food manufacturers and large supermarket chains launched advertising campaigns, pushing certain products and influencing the population's eating habits. For example, breakfast was heavily promoted as one of the most important meals of the day and gradually hundreds of products appeared on the shelves to satisfy this concept. Today, there are dozens of offers of different varieties of cereals on the supermarket shelves, all loaded with sugar (HFCS) and preservatives which all contribute to the diabetes crisis and several other killer diseases. They have almost no nutritional value. According to one study, supermarkets have managed to increase our average daily intake of calories from 3,200 in the 80's to more than 3,900 today, mostly with sugar.

To make things worse, a new industry emerged to resolve this new "overweight" problem - the dieting industry. Today, this is also a billion dollar movement pushing all types of concepts to ostensibly help people lose the weight they put on buying products which were not healthy for them in the first place. We have all tried a diet at some point in our lives and some of us more than one. What happened? We started with all good intentions only to give up at some point and put back the pounds we lost plus a few more. The problem is, we tried to change the way we eat but the world around us didn't change! Supermarkets were still refining their methods to convince us to eat products that are not healthy.

As a non-regulated industry, the sellers of diets can claim almost anything they want and show before-and-after pictures of people who have used their dieting solution. In the majority of cases these pictures come from one of the stock photo providers and the individuals are just models, not actual dieters. If one compares many of these diets, they can often be contradictory to each other, pushing either high or low carbs, high or low fat, with or without protein or various combinations of all of them. In many cases they are not healthy and in some cases outright dangerous.

So now we come back to fasting. Who is going to push, advertise and promote this concept? Nobody and no company is going to make any money if you decide to follow my plan and fast for 90 days. On the contrary, almost all of the present players in the food and health industries risk losing revenue and therefore profits. All they have is irrational arguments why you shouldn't at least give it a try.

My answer is **"The Trial Of ONE"**. You have nothing to lose and it costs you nothing so give it a try. OK, you may have spent a couple of bucks buying my book but, as I explained, this is an investment in yourself you will probably make it back in one day through the money you will save on food!

Opposing Forces - The Government

How on earth could the Government be against **Intermittent Fasting**? Well, let's think about this for a minute. In the previous two chapters we have been talking about two things - (1) The cost to the economy of illness in the population as a whole and (2) The tremendous financial impact on all the jobs and revenue contributors of the "illness industry".

These include the food processing industry, the supermarket chains together with their distribution networks, all the healthcare providers from your family doctor to the clinics and hospitals, the suppliers of equipment and technology to these segments, the pharmaceutical industry with their research facilities, to a lesser extent the dieting and nutritional supplement industry and all the other support institutions from universities, building contractors, tax and finance institutions, insurance companies and even government employees counting and managing all the tax dollars that originate from all of these activities. Last but not least, we have the poor consumers who work in these industries who pay taxes on their income to both the State and Federal Governments.

So, even though the government could save the billions they spend on healthcare each and every year, the amount of money they make from the taxes the Illness Industry creates far outweighs these savings. During the course of reading this book, maybe you will begin to understand the enormous impact a nationwide **Intermittent Fasting** campaign could have on our society. BTW, this was my main motivation in writing this book - to spread the word.

The only institution that could launch such a nationwide education program would be the government. To test any theory, I have always used the "extreme case scenario" to prove a case. The extreme case scenario here would be the government to issue a nationwide decree that every citizen be obliged to implement at least three **Intermittent Fasting** periods each and every year. I know this will never happen but let's just look at the pros and the cons if it did.

What would be the effect on the population? We would eat less, reduce obesity, live a much healthier life with fewer illnesses, improve our body's ability to deal with stress and postpone or even eliminate diseases like cancer, cardiovascular diseases, diabetes, Alzheimer's and Parkinson's to mention just a few. These are the pros.

What are the cons? The food industry would experience a reduction in revenue and profits, supermarkets would have to close some stores, doctors and hospitals would have fewer customers, Big Pharma would sell fewer drugs, the dieting industry would go out of business and all of the professionals and industries supporting these segments of the economy would suffer financial setbacks. To make things worse, we would all live a lot longer which would put a tremendous pressure on retirement plans.

This is looking at the pros and cons from a logical standpoint. From the Government's point of view I would have to switch the pros and cons. Although such a drastic measure would benefit the population as a whole, for the Government it would result in a drastic cut in tax revenue on which it thrives. To make sure it will not happen, all of these industry players have such a lobbying impact on the government, they will make sure the status quo stays intact.

Therefore, once you have fasted and proven to yourself that it works, it is imperative **YOU** spread the word and maybe share this book (and others) with your friends and family. This is the ONLY way the concept of **Intermittent Fasting** will spread and how all of us can take control of our own destiny, claim back our health and live a healthier, longer life.

3. DISCOVERY

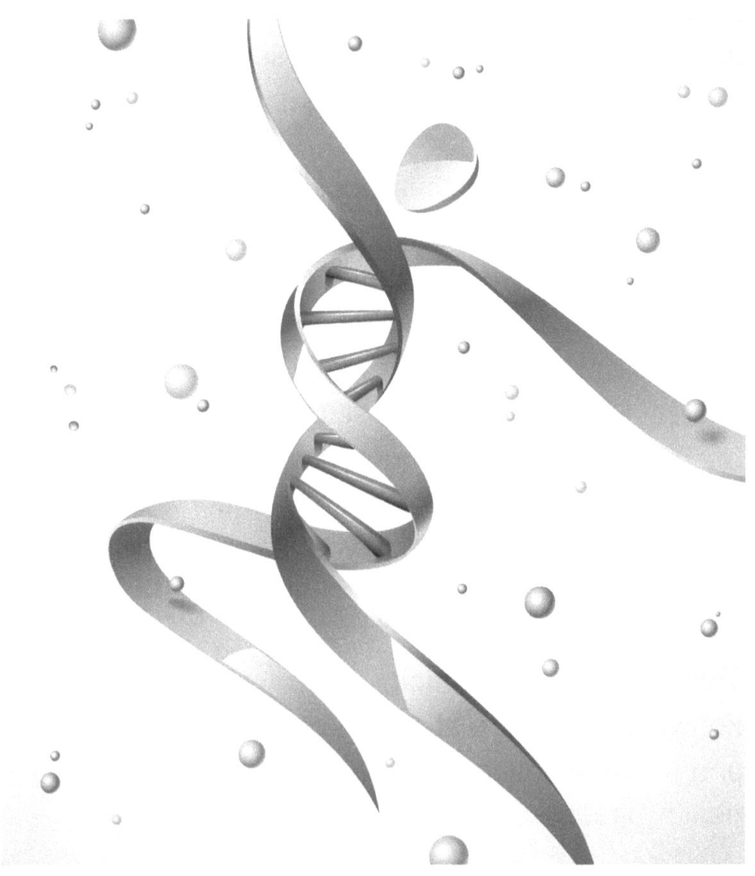

It's Not Your Fault

This is a phrase we can read in almost all the publications dealing with weight loss and dieting. When it comes to being overweight, it cannot be farther from the truth! I once visited a seminar by the famous motivator, Zig Ziglar where he was addressing the issue of weight loss and he posed this question to one of his overweight participants:

"Did you ever eat anything accidentally?" - Zig Ziglar

The answer is obvious but it resides at the core of the problem. We are at the mercy of our environment and lack the basic education as to how we can maintain a healthy lifestyle and avoid all these diseases. In all of my years at school I cannot remember one course on nutrition and health. All I can remember is my mother telling me "you are what you eat" as she tried to guide me on the right track.

This creates a situation where, without any basic knowledge, we are at the mercy of our environment and outside influences when it comes to living a healthy lifestyle.

If we take a look first at the food industry, and here I also include supermarkets and restaurants, its main interest is feeding us as much food as possible and making as much profit as possible. If we look at supermarkets, they have managed to increase our average daily intake of calories from 3,200 in the 80's to more than 3,900 today. More food, more profits. To make things worse, the food processing industry has discovered cheaper ingredients to reduce their manufacturing costs and increase profits, often with ingredients that are bad for our health.

One of those has been the introduction of High Fructose Corn Syrup (HFCS), a highly sweet by-product of waste corn. This is incredibly inexpensive and has become the sweetener of choice for the food manufacturers. To make things worse, scientist now believe that HFCS is addictive and entices us to eat more. Good for shareholders, bad for consumers.

Eating out has also changed. Gone are the days when we used to go to the local family restaurant serving fresh food and dined out with people we knew. Now we have become franchised. This is an environment where business interests prevail, everything is standardized and restaurant chains focus on reducing their costs of ingredients. The local coffee shop is now Starbucks, the local sandwich shop Subway, the local diner Denny's and the exotic night out is Chipotle. Prices are reasonable, the servings are big and the nutritional content questionable. This is a guaranteed highway to obesity!

So what can you do about this? A simple answer could be: Stop eating! The real answer is a little more complex. What is clear, the core of the answer is that **YOU** have to take control. Waiting for the government to create some kind of regulation of the food industry to benefit your health is not going to happen. One of the purposes of this book is to provide you with information and solutions to either avoid becoming overweight or obese in the first place or escape from it as quickly as possible and stay slim and healthy. We have all been programmed to believe weight loss is an uphill battle which most of us lose. This is a myth we have to change.

But the first step is **YOU**. **Intermittent Fasting** is a simple method of fasting for you to lose the weight you want, to keep it off, to replenish the cells in your body, to avoid most of the deadly diseases you might suffer from, to create a more confident and productive you and to do this **FOR FREE!** But it is up to you and the one thing I cannot control is your mindset. This has to be **your part of the deal**. The decision to do it is yours. Therefore, probably the most important chapter in his book is the the one entitled "Motivation", as it describes the preparation work that only you can do. Please read it carefully more than once!

Path Of Discovery

Someone once said that everything starts as an idea or an inspiration. Well, in my case this book started as a conviction, a conviction that we have solutions to our problems within our own control. It is so easy to blame someone or something else for all the negative things that could happen to us. I could list a number of examples of this but instead I want to focus on just one aspect of your life you can individually control...this is your health.

Being alive is one of the best things that could have happened to us and I believe it is our duty to make the best out of the time we have on this planet. There is a starting date and an end date and I have always wondered what people might think of me when I'm gone, in particular family and friends. We all have memories of people we knew who have left us. Are they positive or negative? What will people be thinking of you when you are no longer with us?

This question led me to think of my grandchildren and my own children. What might they think of me when I'm gone? One problem is I waited too long before starting my family so now, in my early seventies, my grandchildren have only recently been born and are still young. Using elementary maths, I suddenly realized that if I am not careful they might not even remember their grandad! Now we cannot normally choose the moment when we leave this life but we have the power to influence it. This brings me back to the question of your health.

I recently went through major heart surgery to replace my aortic valve for the second time, something I knew was coming, but it was still something that made me pause and wonder how much longer I will be here. Will I be able to experience the graduation of any of my grandkids? To answer yes to this question I will have to live at least another 15 years or so which will take me into my late eighties. Now, I could just wait, believe in fate, and see what happens, or take steps that increase my chances of being the grandad my grandchildren might remember. These thoughts led me to the question of fasting, but I will have to fill in the blanks.

I believe I have lived a fairly healthy life. Always included sport in my routine, have never smoked, drink in moderation and don't take unnecessary risks. Visits to doctors have always been a rare event and even when I was sick, have always looked towards alternatives to swallowing medicines. During the 20 years I lived in North America I consulted with naturopathic doctors and not MD's. Around 2005 I was introduced to a company by the name of LifeVantage and a product called Protandim. This is not the subject of this book but it introduced me to a new branch of science by the name of Nutrigenomics.

Nutrigenomics is the study of how things we ingest have an impact on our genetic pathways. The emergence of this new science has been made possible by the incredible advancements in technology which now allow scientists to study and understand what happens in our bodies at the micro-molecular level. This has become the biggest threat to the global pharmaceutical industry as it is discovering new ways we can cure ailments and diseases with simple plant extracts and not medicines. In some cases it is setting conventional wisdom on its head.

I used to think we are born with a particular combination of the genetic code which determines our character and many other things including our health. How often have we heard that some people are more genetically inclined to contract a particular disease because "it runs in the family". Some people actually believe our date of death is somehow magically programmed into this code. Modern science and research has now proven this not to be the case. Scientists now know how the human genome works and how it can be influenced by the things we eat. Welcome to Nutrigenomics!

I have been taking Protandim now for more than ten years as I believe science has proven it protects my body from the dangerous effects free radicals have on my cells. During this time I have immersed myself in the research on molecular biology now taking place on how our bodies function and survive. This led me online to a film produced by the BBC called "Fasting in North America" where a reporter did some research on fasting by putting himself through a number of fasting programs in the USA, under medical supervision. I had heard about fasting before but only in connection with different religions and people who do it to detoxify their bodies.

Although I had no idea what fasting actually was, I assumed it was a process of putting the body through some method of starvation which I immediately connected with something unpleasant. It summoned up the terrible pictures of starving children in Africa and other developing countries. How could starving the body and hunger do any good? In fact it must damage the body which is designed to accept food and nourish itself, right? Well, I was wrong which brings me back again to my conviction and motivation about controlling my health and living longer.

The BBC film set me on a path of discovery. Since then I have read hundreds of research studies, watched dozens of films, experienced my own fasts and met lots of people who have done the same and I am here to tell you that fasting provides a method of avoiding many of the diseases we die from as well as allowing us to live a more active, more satisfying life. My interest in fasting has provided me with a possible method and a path to live healthier and longer. I cannot help but think of many famous people who lived very long lives. I don't believe any of them were overweight and suffering from diabetes. They were almost always slim. Mother Theresa and Gandhi just come to mind. In fact, nobody comes directly to mind who lived to a hundred who was overweight.

Modern science has now discovered what actually happens to our bodies at the molecular level when we deprive it of food and it is something the rest of the medical industry doesn't want you to know.

Although fasting is something the human race has been doing for thousands of years, modern research on the subject is still in its infancy. One reason is that companies and/or industries are not interested in funding research that puts them out of business. The billions of dollars invested on this planet in medical research is invested in discovering how to treat diseases, not how to avoid them. In fact, all pharmaceutical companies are in the business of treating diseases, not preventing them. Taking an aspirin has never resolved the problem of having a headache. To make things even worse, governments accept the lobbying contributions of Big Pharma which impacts election campaigns and encourages governments to take decisions and pass legislation which only benefits them. In many western countries governments are also the biggest single customer of the Pharma Industry.

So who is carrying out this new research? There are a number of academic scientists who are the banner holders of these ideas and who are being funded mainly by private foundations. However, as the word starts to spread, momentum is beginning to build and people are starting their own fasting plan and telling others about the incredible benefits they have experienced. This "word-of-mouth" advertising, including books like this, are beginning to have a major impact on the spread of this concept. The good news is doing a fast costs you nothing. In fact you actually save money as you will probably be eating less!

As this book is "A Beginner's Guide" I do not address every single fasting plan such as the severe and long-term fasting plans that can involve not eating for weeks or months. These are mostly conducted under medical supervision and often have specific medical goals. I address **Intermittent Fasting Plans** that are easy to understand, easy to implement and are adjustable based on your own personal preferences. The motivation to start a your fast is addressed in the Chapter "Motivation" but briefly the most common goal is to lose weight. Fasting is not a diet, it is a change in lifestyle. It is a focus on what you feed your body and when you eat.

This also puts the dieting industry at risk. My research forced me to take a look at the huge number of diets that are being advertised and for which consumers are laying out billions of dollars each and every year. In fact almost everyone has tried some sort of diet with the promise of losing those extra pounds. The common element of most diets is they don't work! After painstakingly following the diet, we give up and put those extra pounds back on plus a few more. Interestingly enough, a number of studies have tried to prove that calorie restriction (typical with diets) is as effective as fasting, all funded by the diet industry! This is a sure sign the dieting community is concerned about the threat of fasting.

As I became more knowledgeable about how my body functions, I was amazed at some of the claims the dieting industry is making. Incredible before and after pictures with promises of losing pound upon pound, day after day. Fortunately, the Internet allows us to check out some of these offers and I discovered that most of the before and after pictures were not real people but pictures acquired from stock photo providers. This is why I took some simple, very amateurish videos of my first serious fast. These have not been altered in Photoshop and show the real results of the fasting plan I recommend.

So, although I have no formal medical qualifications, I have studied the writings of almost every expert in this field and my own personal conviction forced me to write this book to make you aware of a method by which you can:

- Lose weight quickly and safely

- A way to keep off the fat and maintain a healthy weight

- Change your attitude towards nutrition

- Have the potential to live a longer life

- Repair and renew the cellular structure of your body

- Understand the dangers of consuming pharmaceutical medications

- Avoid many of the diseases people die from

- Make you aware of how your body functions

- Give you more confidence and a greater mental focus

- Save money

- Take the decision to include fasting as part of your life

I recommend that you take the time to watch the films and read some of the articles that I have included as links at the end of the book so that you can also be as convinced as I am. They represent months of intensive research on the subject and, as it was with me, your own conviction will be the basis of your success. There will be enough naysayers in your direct environment and people who think you are crazy to "starve" yourself to good health. But you will overcome this challenge and be a motivator of others. This will be the way the concept of fasting will spread and become mainstream. Become a **Trial of ONE**! Here's to your success!

The Fight Against Fat

I think that most experts now agree that body fat is a killer. It has proven to be the main cause of many of the lethal diseases that we die from. Whether it be cardiovascular diseases, diabetes, many forms of cancer or even Alzheimer's, scientists have discovered that being overweight can and will lead to your death.

One of the questions I have always pondered is why then do we become obese and overweight in the first place? Looking at the evolution of mankind, it is a relatively new phenomenon. In ages past, the problem was the exact reverse. Where will our next meal come was the biggest concern. When will the hunter in the family slaughter the next animal so we can eat? In fact, even today, in many parts of the world the problem is gaining weight, not losing it. In many countries in Africa, if you carry around extra fat you are regarded to be one of the affluent few.

So, why do we gain weight in the first place? The main reason is that in our modern society, food consumption has gone from a necessity to survive to a full-blown industry with shareholders who want to make a profit. We are now bombarded with advertisements selling products that are full of calories, drenched in fat, enhanced with sugar and all produced in a factory using chemicals that are bad for us. Then we buy these products in huge supermarkets, which entice us through the aisles with offers to satisfy the appetite of our tastebuds and not our need to live a healthier life. Then they sell and advertise food with substances that make them even more addictive.

To make things worse, the food industry has circulated misinformation about eating in general. "Eat at least three meals every day" or "Breakfast is the most important meal in the day" are typical expressions that have been promoted by the food industry but debunked by the latest research.

Moreover, we now have access to technologies and vehicles which encourage us to be less active. We are sitting almost all day long. Whether we are in front of the television, driving our car or tipping away on our smartphones, our bodies are not being programmed to burn calories. In fact we often look for the parking space closest to the supermarket to go buy our junk food rather than the space farthest away with the most exercise.

Of course, we never run out of excuses. Getting older, having to raise a family, the importance of our career as well as the need to relax in this stressful world always seems to lead to less exercise. Most families have two cars in the garage, but no bikes and even if they have bikes, they almost never use them. Going for a walk in the evening is no longer part of our culture. In fact in many cities today there are no sidewalks any more. I was once in a hotel in New Jersey and got up early to go for a jog only to discover there was no path or sidewalk to jog on.

So here we are, getting older and slowly putting on more weight each week, every month and every year, almost unnoticed. It only becomes a problem when we go out to buy new clothes. Our pants or the dress size doesn't quite fit any more so we just take a size bigger and live with that for another year. Suddenly we are overweight. Sitting in front of our television we are shown advertisements for the latest diets or devices to magically make our abs appear. We might not be terribly impressed but then one of our friends or family members tells us about this great weight loss program they are following.

At this point, and this can occur at any age, we experience the first signs of doubt about the life we are leading. This is the first stage of a guilty conscience. Being overweight leads to heart disease, diabetes and even cancer! Alcohol and smoking lead to addiction and maybe an early death. Maybe we believe more exercise is the answer and we go online and order a treadmill or some weights. Perhaps joining a gym is the answer. After all, just doing a few of those „abs exercises" will bring back the six-pack, right? Then our guilty conscience gets to us and we start our first diet either because our partner decides to do it or because we believe the evidence and the before and after pictures are so overwhelming, it must be true.

We cut out carbs, or fat, or protein or eat more of this and less of that, start exercising more and begin to acquire the bathroom scale fever. We jump on the scale when we wake up in the morning and before going to bed at night. We start taking notes of our progress. Maybe we join Weight Watchers or an online program. Then there are the latest "scientific discoveries" that propose taking a certain pill and the pounds will just roll off. The weight-loss Industry is born. It makes billions of dollars preying on our guilty consciences and convincing us that handing over, or investing, a few bucks every month will solve our weight problems.

Months later, we come to the conclusion that this dieting thing is just too complicated and we give up. We succumb again to all the old temptations and routines that got us into this state in the first place. We put back all the pounds that we lost plus a few more and become non-believers in the world of fitness/wellness. The treadmill and weights start to collect dust in the garage and are sold off at the next garage sale. We cover ourselves with all sorts of excuses. "Tried that and it didn't work" or "Will add it to my next New Year's Resolutions". This has created an unhealthy, obese, fat nation! Are you one of them?

The Fat You Cannot See

If you are somewhat overweight and take a look in the mirror then you can probably see the fat causing the problem. But that is not the problem. The problem is all the fat you cannot see, accumulating inside of your body around your most important organs such as your heart, liver and kidneys. This fat is known as visceral fat.

Visceral fat is technically excess intra-abdominal fat accumulation. In other words, it's known as a "deep" fat that's stored further underneath the skin than the belly fat you can see. It's a form of gel-like fat that's actually wrapped around your major internal organs. If you have a protruding belly and large waist, that's a clear sign you are storing dangerous, visceral fat. While it's most noticeable and pronounced in obese individuals, anyone can have visceral fit, many without even knowing it.

Visceral fat is especially dangerous because these fat cells do more than just sit there and cause your pants to feel tight — they also change the way your body operates. Modern science has now proven that excess visceral fat can often be the cause of a number of problematic reactions. Here are some of them:

1. <u>Increased Inflammation</u>

A major concern is that visceral fat produces hormonal and inflammatory molecules that get dumped directly into the liver, leading to even more inflammation and hormone-disrupting reactions. If you have more fat stored than you need, especially around organs like the liver, heart and kidneys, your body becomes inflamed and your metabolism suffers, making it a hard to break the cycle.

Visceral fat does more than just lead to inflammation down the road — it becomes inflamed itself by producing something known as interleukin-6, a type of inflammatory molecule. This type of fat stores inflammatory white blood cells and kicks off a series of autoimmune reactions. Inflammation is the root cause of most diseases, and this is why inflammatory belly fat is linked with cognitive decline, arthritis, cancer, diabetes and so on. It is also the reason I take the product I have already mentioned - Protandim.

2. <u>Higher Risk of Diabetes</u>

More than other types of fats, visceral fat is known to play a role in insulin resistance, which means a heightened risk for developing diabetes. For example, abdominal fat is viewed as a bigger health risk than hip or thigh fat, not only for diabetes but for many other chronic diseases.

While men are more likely to store noticeable levels of visceral fat, women are also greatly at risk. Reducing visceral fat through **Intermittent Fasting** is one of the most important natural diabetes treatments which is totally under your control.

3. Makes It Harder to Lose Weight

People tend to get heavier and heavier as time goes on and one of the main reasons is stored body fat affects hunger levels, especially visceral fat. It might seem hard to imagine, but your metabolism is largely governed by your level of existing stored fat. Fat messes with your appetite and makes it easier for you to overeat due to hormonal changes that take place.

Higher levels of insulin also promote more efficient conversion of our calories into body fat, so this becomes a vicious cycle. Eating refined carbohydrates in processed food, as opposed to complex carbohydrates in their natural state like vegetables and fruit, can cause the body's "set point" for body weight to increase. Your "set point" is basically the weight that your body tries to maintain through control of the brain's hormonal messengers.

When you eat refined carbohydrates such as white flour and sugar, the fat-storing hormones are produced in excess, raising the set point and making it harder to follow a healthy diet. This is why it's important to stop your sugar addiction and address weight gain and visceral fat early on, as opposed to letting the situation escalate and become a problem.

4. <u>Higher Risk for Heart Disease and Strokes</u>

Fat-generated inflammation is one of the main contributors to heart disease and other inflammatory disorders. When your body is inflamed, your liver becomes overwhelmed with cholesterol and toxins, which leads to plaque buildup in your arteries. Visceral fat is also associated with an increased risk for cardiovascular disease markers like high triglycerides, high blood pressure and high cholesterol.

5. <u>More Likely to Cause Dementia</u>

A growing body of evidence points to the fact that there's a strong link between obesity, vascular disease, inflammation and cognitive decline, including dementia. In fact, there appears to be a connection between excess pounds and less brain volume and, therefore, poorer brain function as we age.

Research shows people with the biggest bellies have a higher risk of dementia than those with smaller bellies. This is even true even for people with excess belly fat but who overall have a normal weight! The bigger the belly the more negative impact felt on the brain's memory center.

Results from a 2010 study done by the Department of Cardiology at Oita Red Cross Hospital in Japan found that elevated levels of visceral fat in non-dementia patients with type 2 diabetes is characterized by abnormal changes in brain volume and insulin resistance. Other studies have also found that people with belly fat have a higher risk for small strokes, which are particularly associated with declining brain function.

6. <u>Higher Likelihood to Have Depression and Mood Problems</u>

Since excess body fat is linked to hormonal changes and other brain neurotransmitters, excess body fat can negatively impact your mood.

A 2014 study conducted by Boston University School of Medicine found that depressive symptoms are associated with visceral fat in middle-aged adults. To examine the relationship between measures of visceral fat and depression, researchers examined visceral fat tissue and depressive symptoms in 1,581 women (mean age 52.2 years) and 1,718 men (mean age 49.8 years).

After adjusting for age, body mass index, smoking, alcohol and other factors, results showed that higher levels of stored visceral fat translated to higher likelihood of experiencing depression. Other studies show, this fat is a unique pathogenic fat that consists of metabolically active adipose tissue that interferes with healthy brain function.

Depression is especially associated with greater fat storage in women, so it might be even more crucial for women to burn visceral fat. In a study of middle-aged women over 50 years of age, visceral fat, but not visible belly fat or waist circumference, was related to depressive symptoms.

All in all, there are tons of reasons why we should be taking the risk of visceral fat seriously. The crazy thought is, all we have to do to get rid of this problem is to get on the **Intermittent Fasting Plan** I propose and just skip one meal per day. That's it. It is totally free and easy to do. Plus there is tons of other evidence what **Intermittent Fasting** can achieve for your health. The only reason you haven't yet experienced a fast is probably because you haven't heard about it before. There is nobody out there selling this concept because actually there is nothing to sell...**it's FREE**! If you are now convinced, go to Chapter 5 and start your plan.

The Muscles You Cannot See

Millions of men at some time in their lives have been motivated to purchase the latest diet, join a health club or buy some type of sports apparatus for the home. One of the most convincing parts of the promotion is the before and after photos which show what our "six-pack" abs will look like if we just follow the instructions. They somehow represent the virile male we all want to be. But as we have all discovered, it just isn't that easy.

The problem is this. Our six-pack is covered with the belly fat we carry around with us and in order to be able to see these abs, we have to lose this belly fat first. No matter how long you train the ab muscles, if you are overweight, you will never see them. To make things worse, even if you do train your abs hard, it is impossible to target fat loss to any one part of the body through training. Fat loss occurs gradually over the whole body. In fact, one of the last places fat will disappear is around your six-pack! Forget all those claims from equipment manufacturers who entice us with pictures athletes with the perfect six-pack. They often don't have once ounce of fat on them!

So the only efficient way to "reveal" your abs is through fasting, not exercise. In fact, with fat loss your abs (yes you do have some) will magically start appearing even without abs training. This brings to me the statues we sometimes see of the ancient Roman and Greek gods. All of them have incredible bodies and in particular a washboard of abs. Did they have access to modern Sport Club equipment and perform sit-ups every day? Probably not but they were also not eating processed junk food and were probably fasting occasionally.

The Sugar Demon

If I had to pick just one threat to our overall health and the main cause of being overweight, I would have to choose sugar. There are, of course, good and bad sugars. Sugar that exists in naturally occurring foods such as fruit and some vegetables, if not consumed in excess, can be good for us. I am talking about ALL the other sugars that are used to enhance taste and, in some cases, to create addiction. Yes, I did write ADDICTION.

In modern times the population just in the USA has gone from consuming about **20 teaspoons** of sugar per person per year to **150 pounds of sugar** per person per year. That's about half a pound each day for every man, woman and child! In such volumes sugar becomes toxic. But how is this possible?

In almost all processed foods there is an over-abundance of sugar which manufacturers include to enhance the taste. The problem here is they are not even using natural sugar (from sugar cane) but a fructose sugar that has been manufactured from corn starch. The complete name is actually High Fructose Corn Syrup (HFCS). This HFCS is a big danger to your health. Without going into a long medical explanation here, it suffices to say that it leads to a fatty liver, pre-diabetes, Type 2 diabetes and subsequently heart attacks, stroke, cancer and dementia.

HFCS is also one of the main culprits for your weight gain. Your liver doesn't have a chance to process all the sugar you feed it so it converts the majority of it into fat which is then stored in your fat cells. Unhealthy weight gain. Many studies have been published on the detrimental impact HFCS has on your body and still the food industry lobbies with all its power to avoid the public finding out about this tragedy. This battle always focuses on what has to be disclosed on processed food product labels and to make sure you are not able to take your own, informed decision on what is good for your health, the true amount of HFCS is not disclosed. It is just called "sugar".

Do you want to avoid contracting cancer in your life? Then make sure you don't consume too much sugar and HFCS. Although there is competing evidence whether too much sugar intake can cause cancer to develop, there is no doubt that fat or obese people develop cancer much more than people who have a normal weight. A simple solution is to avoid consuming as many processed foods as possible and focus your eating on products that are fresh or at least with ingredients you can understand. At the end of this book we give you some ideas on what to eat when you are at home and also when you are eating out.

4. THE SCIENCE

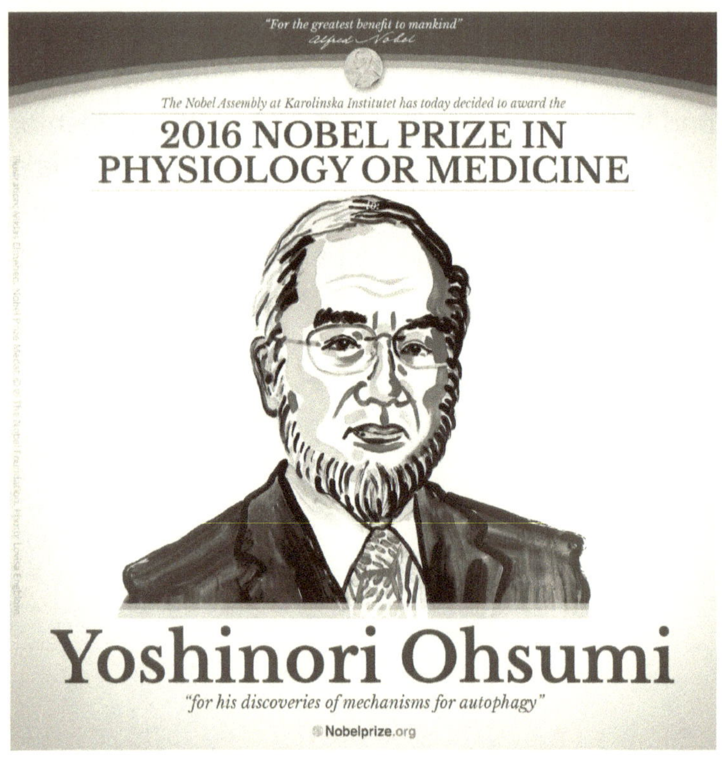

The Science Behind Intermittent Fasting

Fasting has been around for centuries but **Intermittent Fasting** is a relatively new phenomenon. It came to the forefront when it was discovered that many of the benefits of longer-term fasting could still be achieved when one fasted in short intervals (intermittently). It is a little-known fact that a lot of the initial research on longer-term fasting and its effect on health was carried out in Russia. In the 1920's there were clinics in Siberia testing various forms of longer-term fasting and its impact on patients' health. At the end of this book you will find a link to a website that contains a film about this initial research carried out by the Russians.

With the rapid development of technology, it has now enabled scientists and researchers to study what really happens in the human body at the micro-cellular level. The mapping of the human genome is an example of this. Scientists have begun to understand what happens in human cells, how the various processes work and how we can influence them. There are many major processes in our bodies that are activated by **Intermittent Fasting** and they have now been studied and well documented:

1. Autophagy - The Repair Unit

2. Ketosis - The Fat Burner

3. Ghrelin, the Hunger Hormone

4. Insulin, the Sugar Hormone

5. BDNF - The Brain's Fertilizer

Let's take a look at each of them:

1. Autophagy - The Repair Unit

Autophagy has been one of the major discoveries that have been made in the past decade in understanding how our bodies (cells) deal with diseases and the aging process. In 2016 a Japanese scientist by the name of Yoshinori Ohsumi was awarded the Nobel Prize for Medicine for the work and discoveries in this important segment of medicine. Here is an excerpt from the citation issued by the Nobel Prize Committee:

"Thanks to Ohsumi and others following in his footsteps, we now know that autophagy controls important physiological functions where cellular components need to be degraded and recycled. Autophagy can rapidly provide fuel for energy and building blocks for renewal of cellular components, and is therefore essential for the cellular response to

starvation and other types of stress. After infection, autophagy can eliminate invading intracellular bacteria and viruses. Autophagy contributes to embryo development and cell differentiation. Cells also use autophagy to eliminate damaged proteins and organelles, a quality control mechanism that is critical for counteracting the negative consequences of aging".

In other words, autophagy is a renewal process of the cells the body undertakes where it cleans out the junk of damaged structures, reprocesses them for reuse and then discards and eliminates the rest. The really good news is that **Intermittent Fasting is one of the fastest and most efficient methods of kickstarting the autophagy process**, something conventional diets can never lay claim to.

Moreover, you are not awarded a Nobel Prize for anything unless it is for researching and discovering something that provides a major benefit for mankind.

2. Ketosis - The Fat Burner

Normally the body gets its energy from glucose (sugar) and sometimes protein. This glucose comes from eating food with carbohydrates (carbs) which is transferred into the blood stream as glucose. As we eat at least three meals per day and then have snacks in between, there is a constant supply of glucose being provided to the body. Any excess glucose we don't use is then converted and stored as fat.

However, the human body has a backup method of creating energy should the source of glucose be reduced and/or be completely depleted. Our emergency backup reserves for energy are stored in our fat cells and ketosis is the process the body uses to access this fat. Ketones are produced and enter the blood stream and become the source the body can burn for energy. What scientists have discovered is that ketones are the preferred and more efficient source of energy for different parts of our body. This is partly the reason you will feel an extreme sense of extra energy and mental sharpness once you are more than a week into your **Intermittent Fast**.

It is true that during the beginning of your **Intermittent Fast** you may suffer from some headaches and light-headiness but this has nothing to do with ketosis and more with your body adjusting to this new environment.

Science has already established that ketones are a much more efficient source for energy than glucose (sugar). They are also recognized as a neuroprotective antioxidant which provides many other substantial benefits including the potential for preventing and reversing brain damage related to such conditions as epilepsy, autism and Parkinson's disease, something I have already touched upon.

Here is a limited summary of some of the key benefits of using ketones, created through **Intermittent Fasting**, as an alternative source for energy:

A. Weight Loss

- the quickest and most efficient method of burning excess fat
- Insulin levels drop dramatically

B. Blood Sugar Control

- Fasting automatically lowers levels of blood sugar
- Can prevent or eliminate Type 2 diabetes

C. Lower Blood Pressure & Cholesterol

- Blood pressure benefits from decreased weight
- Improved Cholesterol levels and Triglycerides

D. Insulin Resistance

- Can lower insulin levels dramatically
- Prevent or even cure Type 2 diabetes (medical supervision recommended).

These benefits and more are achieved with **Intermittent Fasting**.

3. Ghrelin - The Hunger Hormone

One of the main fears that you may have when it comes to starting an **Intermittent Fasting** program is the hunger you can expect to suffer. The hunger feeling is caused by the hormone ghrelin (I call it the hunger gremlin!). It is released into your blood stream by the stomach, travels to the brain to signal "I am hungry"! You WILL experience some strong hunger feelings at the beginning of your **Intermittent Fasting** plan but they will decrease over time. The vast majority of people I have talked to (including myself!), confirm that after day three of the fast this hunger feeling subsides and the hunger gremlin leaves you alone.

This absence of ghrelin has many other positive effects. Not only does it help in the fasting process itself by eliminating the sudden need to succumb to temptation and break the fast, it also takes away the need to overeat during your eating period. In my case, what I find interesting is the hunger hormone has never returned, even though my **Intermittent Fasting** plan ended more than three months ago. I can honestly say that the reason I now eat is because

I want to and not because I am hungry. This has eliminated the yo-yo effect and has allowed me to maintain my newly won body.

BTW, as a side note, the disappearance of the hunger gremlin is not achieved by any of the other weight loss dieting programs.

4. Insulin - The Sugar Hormone

During digestion, foods that contain carbohydrates (sugar) are converted into glucose. Most of this glucose is sent into your bloodstream, causing a rise in blood glucose levels. This increase in blood glucose signals your pancreas to produce insulin.

The insulin tells cells throughout your body to take in glucose from your bloodstream. As the glucose moves into your cells, your blood glucose levels go down. Some cells use the glucose as energy. Other cells, such as in your liver and muscles, store any excess glucose as a substance called glycogen. Your body uses glycogen for fuel between meals.

In the event we consume more carbohydrates, and therefore more glucose, than the body can absorb in energy, insulin converts these into fat and stores them around the body in our fat cells. What often happens over time though, these excesses of glucose in the body can help develop a resistance to insulin. In other words, the body no longer believes in the signal and doesn't produce enough insulin and the body sugar levels start to increase.

In insulin resistance, muscle, fat, and liver cells do not respond properly to insulin and therefore cannot easily absorb glucose from the bloodstream. As a result, the body needs even higher levels of insulin to promote a response for glucose to enter our cells and diabetes develops where patients inject more insulin into their bloodstream.

Over time, insulin resistance can lead to type 2 diabetes and pre-diabetes because the beta cells fail to keep up with the body's increased need for insulin. Without enough insulin, excess glucose builds up in the bloodstream, leading to diabetes, pre-diabetes, and other serious health disorders.

The standard cure for type 2 diabetes is to inject more insulin into the body either in tablet form or directly into the bloodstream but this leads to a vicious cycle and doesn't solve the problem. The insulin resistance increases, more fat is stored and obesity begins.

Scientists have now discovered that a better way to burn off the excess sugars (glucose) in our bodies is to fast. As the need for insulin declines, the body turns for its energy needs to ketone bodies and the process of ketosis begins (see above).

Several well-renowned doctors and scientists are now trying to promote fasting as the ultimate solution to both prevent and cure type 2 diabetes, which is known as one of the biggest killer diseases of our generation. Of course, Big Pharma will do everything in its power to resist this change as its involves billions of dollars of income and profits for them.

5. BDNF - Your Brain's Fertilizer

BDNF stands for Brain Derived Neurotrophic Factor and is a powerful little protein that stimulates your production of new brain cells and strengthens existing ones. More specifically, when you release BDNF, it flips the switch on of a series of genes that grow brand new brain cells and pathways. High BDNF makes you learn faster, remember better, age slower, and rapidly rewires your brain.

BDNF also increases your brain's plasticity. When your brain cells get damaged or face a stressful situation, BDNF protects them and helps them come back stronger. Your neural pathways become more flexible instead of shutting down, which could explain why higher levels of BDNF are associated with warding off depression.

So what does this have to do with **Intermittent Fasting**?

Very recent scientific studies have shown that the quickest and most effective way to activate and create more BDNF is through **Intermittent Fasting**. It is more effective than all the available drugs or physical exercise. In fact, **Intermittent Fasting** has been proven to increase BDNF by up to 400 percent.

Intermittent Fasting holds the key for enhanced brain functioning. It also has very promising evidence on preventing brain degenerative disorders such as Alzheimer's and Parkinson's disease. If you are starting to suffer from memory loss or have ever experienced the so-called "brain fog", then start **Intermittent Fasting** without delay. You have nothing to lose. It is the simplest and cheapest way to enhance the function of your brain.

The Final Analysis

In this chapter we have addressed just a few of the scientific reasons why you should start your **Intermittent Fasting Plan**. There are many more but we cannot address all of them here. There is a large abundance of materials available on the Internet and if this chapter is not enough then I recommend you take the time to do your own research.

The majority of **Intermittent Fasting** proponents approach the subject from purely the weight loss perspective which is fine if that motivates you to give it a try. I have just tried to point out there are also many major health benefits which come for free. Benefits Big Pharma cannot provide. Losing excess fat will certainly make you feel better, look better and become more confident but knowing you are giving your body the chance to repair itself and giving it the tools to avoid many of the diseases modern society suffers from should be just as satisfying. **The best news is it comes for FREE!**

5. MOTIVATION

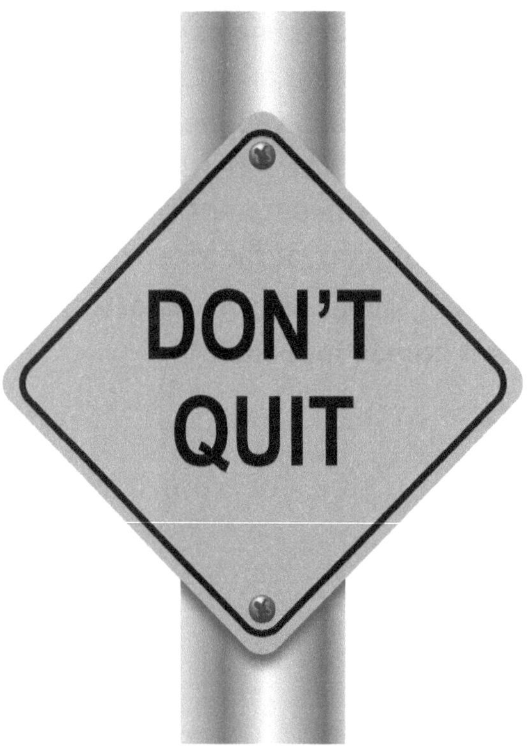

Your Mental Preparation

This is perhaps the most important section in this book. Do not embark on any **Intermittent Fasting Plan** unless you can sincerely answer yes to all five questions at the end of this chapter. The reason why so many weight-loss plans fail is because people pay not enough attention to the subject of commitment at the beginning. It is often just one of the things we routinely add to our list of New Year's Resolutions as an afterthought. But if you embark on a plan designed to avoid major diseases and potentially save your life, then maybe the chances are you might finish it more successfully. If it is just to lose a few pounds, then so many obstacles and excuses will get in the way, you will probably not succeed.

In fact, **Intermittent Fasting** is not a diet, it is a change in your mental attitude towards food and what it can do for you. When you are successful with this plan, you will be leading a completely different life. A life full of things that you didn't imagine were possible. In my case, it took me back about 10 years and gave me a new lease on life, even though I belong to the "Older Generation"! When I think of the 70% of the USA population that is either obese or overweight, I get excited that something so simple and so inexpensive can change so many lives, no matter how old or young you are.

Convincing Yourself

This might sound a bit obvious but I am talking about more than losing just a few pounds or kilos. In my case, I embarked on this journey not to lose wait, but to live a longer life. I have a blog website entitled "Live-Healthier-Longer" where I talk
about how to live a healthier, longer life. Then I stumbled across Michael Mosley's BBC documentary. This introduced me to the subject of fasting which I had heard about but had never taken a closer look at. This peaked my interest to the point where I spent almost every day for the best part of three months reading every article and/or scientific report about fasting that I could find. Some of these articles and reports you will find in the Appendix section at the end of the book and I recommend you read as many as you can.

Then, another good place to start is to watch the film on my website called "The Introduction To Fasting". It is one hour long and I suggest you find the time to watch this film in one single session. Then watch one or more videos from Dr. Valter Longo, the links to which are also located in the Appendix section. Dr. Longo is one of the scientists who is taking the research into fasting to the next level. He explains the problem that nobody or company has any interest in promoting fasting as a solution for obesity or as a cure for the many diseases such as diabetes. There is no money to be made. In fact, fasting is a major threat to the pharmaceutical industry which creates billions in profits keeping people sick and selling them drugs. If diabetes can be cured with fasting, they will lose billions of dollars in revenue.

In Appendix C under the section entitled "Scientific References" are a number of papers which will enhance your understanding of how important fasting has become. You may not be able to understand much of the scientific mumbo jumbo, as I didn't, but you will certainly get the message. Where possible, just read the objectives and then the summaries and conclusions to make it easier. This is an important step to strengthen your own conviction.

If you do any more research on the Internet on the subject of fasting (which you should!) you will come across many naysayers as it completely upsets conventional wisdom and will deprive many of their income. In fact, in one presentation of a certain dieting program they categorically said that fasting can kill you, even though they were promoting a pure protein diet, which if followed too long, could definitely kill you! Nonetheless, there is ample scientific evidence that fasting is a natural phenomenon that has existed and been practiced for thousands of years, not only by humans, but by the whole animal kingdom. It is embedded in our genealogy.

At the end of the day, it is important you not only believe in fasting as a solution to many potential problems, you must develop a strong **DESIRE** to start and finish the plan. I can help you to maintain your progress in our chapters on **MOTIVATION** and there are many tips on how to overcome some of the obstacles you might face after you have started, even though these are few and far between. I encourage you to enjoy your journey of fasting and look forward to the benefits it provides. You will feel you have accomplished something major - which you have!

Prepare Your Environment

The next challenge to address is your environment. Your friends, your family and possibly co-workers. Even though you may have accepted the mission yourself to complete your IF plan, there will be lots of distractions from people around you. They will not have access to the information you have and will not be able to comprehend your mission and the targets you have set. Most of them will think you are just on one of those useless, fad diets that never succeed anyway. They may even relate the word "fasting" to the word "hunger" and see the plan as just another "hunger strike"! You may not have time to explain to them what fasting is all about. In the case of your own family, it could lead to major disruptions as your eating schedule will almost certainly fall outside of the rest of the family's. How should you deal with this problem?

One simple way could be not to even enter into any discussion with anyone during the plan. Don't even try and explain what fasting is all about. Defer every discussion and explanation to the point in time when you have reached your goals so that you can present and discuss concrete results. This will defer any theoretical and vague discussions about what might happen and that the plan cannot be good for you. This is the approach I took with my family when I did my first **Intermittent Fasting Plan**. I tried the path of explaining what I was about to do and finished up in endless, frustrating discussions with family and friends who thought it was all a lot of nonsense and I already looked good anyway! So then I shut up and just executed my plan.

Sometimes people will be negative just because they are jealous. Maybe they would like to try something like this, especially if you show your success, but their own environment will not allow it. During my first fast I finished up being quite alone in order to avoid any type of discourse. This worked out fine as I was able to focus on the plan and my goals and not be distracted by these outside influences. My biggest problem was my own wife, who is an incredible cook, and an important part of her day was preparing fantastic meals for me. I always joke a little about our marriage as the one made in heaven - she loves to cook and I love to eat! But this was suddenly over for a while and it caused some real problems between us. She saw my plan as an invasion into our daily lives.

However, when she saw the progress I was making by simply changing my eating times, she was convinced and she has even joined the cause which makes things a lot easier. So before you start your plan, prepare yourself for such conflicts. It will not only disrupt your own routine but probably that of the people around you. See yourself as a mover and (fat) shaker and as you see the fat melting away you will gain confidence and the problems with your environment will disappear. At that point people will be asking you - what happened?

Setting Goals

One thing I have learned in life is that in order to achieve success in any kind of project, setting goals is always the first step. This is certainly the case with fasting. One of the problems you face is, it is up to you to execute the plan and if you don't succeed you can only blame yourself. Setting goals is an important component to succeed. One overarching goal is you should always adhere to is at least to **finish the plan you started**. This should happen no matter what. At times, it will be so easy to postpone the plan a couple of days or put the plan on hold when things get tough but this will always be seen as a failure, a personal failure.

In my case, I had set a number of goals. Reducing my blood pressure and other markers of my cardiovascular condition were as important as just reducing the fat around my waist. I hate taking medicines and being at the mercy of the pharmaceutical companies. Therefore, achieving this goal would allow me to stop taking the medicines my cardiologist had prescribed for me. Of course, I didn't just do this without consulting her!

Your goals should be clear and definable. Just wishing to lose weight is not enough. Translate losing weight into hard numbers. Is "losing weight" defined as losing a certain number of pounds (or kilos) or perhaps getting into a smaller dress or pant size? In my case, I wanted to go from a jeans size 36" and fit into a jeans size 32" which for me was the absolute measure of how much fat around my middle I could lose. In Europe this would mean going from a size 54 to a size 50. As in this case, your goal(s) should be realistic and measurable. In my case, I could simply try on the pants in my closet!

In some cases it could be beneficial to set interim goals. For those who might be obese or extremely overweight, breaking down the overall goal into smaller, definable steps could be a key to success. For those who are diabetic, continually monitoring blood sugar levels is obviously of key importance and should be a big factor in motivation. However, what is not recommended is stepping on the bathroom scales twice a day. This doesn't count as "interim steps". Your weight will fluctuate from day to day based on what you eat and by your retention or not of fluids

People who go on one of those fad diets often boast about all the weight they are losing in the first week. Unfortunately it is mostly fluids. They already project the first week's weight loss into the future and expect the impossible. This is when they get discouraged and stop the program "because it doesn't work".

One of the keys to completing a successful **Intermittent Fasting Plan** is it must be embedded in your head. If you do not believe that the plan could change **your entire life** for the better and empower you to move on to greater things, then it might not work. The benefits have been extensively proven by science but because fasting is not a profit center for the wellness or healthcare industry, it is often criticized by them. Even your family doctor might not encourage you as it goes against everything he or she studied. Therefore, your self-conviction that it works is the key to your success.

Here are the five questions you should ask yourself and answer honestly:

1. Are you totally convinced of the health benefits of fasting?

2. Have you set your goals and decided how to measure your success?

3. Do you know how to handle objections from your friends and family?

4. Have you decided to finish your program no matter what?

5. At the end, will you share your success with the people around you?

You might consider recording your progress by taking some videos or pictures. I took some videos and have been able to convince other people who have seen them. If you are totally serious keep a diary of the whole event. Write down when and what you ate during your eating period, how you felt every day and what sort of objections and/or reactions you get from people around you. It will be something you can always look back on with pride.

Intermittent Fasting Might Not Be For Some People

Intermittent fasting isn't for everyone. If you belong to any of these categories, talk to your doctor:

- Diabetes 1. If you take anything that regulates your blood sugar levels, then talk to your doctor before considering Intermittent Fasting.

- Eating disorders. Anyone who has any kind of history of or tendency toward anorexia or bulimia should avoid this type of eating as it could trigger a flare-up.

- Pregnant or planning to be pregnant.

- Medications that need to be taken with food. It's possible that you can use some butter or coconut oil to help avoid the discomfort and stomach upset that come when you take some medications on an empty stomach. Alternatively, plan to use the adapted ADF option where breakfast is consumed every day.

6. THE PLAN

PLAN OVERVIEW

TIME	PLAN	ACTION
Step 1 Week 1	Preparation	• Reduce sugar intake • Start sport activity • Follow low-carb diet
Step 2 Weeks 2 - 11	Fast	• 18/6 Fasting Plan • 24/24 Fasting Plan (Alt.) • Select eating plan • Evaluate progress
Step 3 Week 12	Exit	• Evaluate results • Modify eating plan • Establish exit strategy • Decision exit/renew

Your Fasting Plan

If you answered "yes" confidently to all of these five questions, then you are ready to begin your **Intermittent Fasting Plan**.

As I have already mentioned there are two main popular **Intermittent Fasting Plans** which are promoted by many of the experts and these are the so-called 16/8 and 5/2 plans. Either you can choose between an 8-hour window of eating and a 16-hour window of fasting each and every day (16/8) or 5 complete days of eating and 2 complete days of fasting each and every week (5/2). The 16/8 plan, which is the most popular, simply means one has to skip either breakfast or dinner every day.

I decided to modify the 16/8 standard plan into one which I call the 18/6 plan which simply means a 6-hour eating window and an 18-hour fasting window. These extra two hours of fasting compared to the traditional 16/8 plan provides for two more hours of fasting and therefore more ketosis (fat burning) each day, which is when the most fat is being consumed as energy. Over the course of one week this amounts to 14 hours more of ketosis than the 16/8 plan which will have a major impact on your results.

I have also found that adjusting my mealtimes to adapt to an 8-hour eating window (the 16/8 plan) not so convenient. If you eat breakfast at 7.00 am then you would have to eat lunch at the latest by 3.00 pm in the afternoon, which is too late for most people. If you choose to skip breakfast and just eat lunch and dinner then you have the same problem. With a 1.00 pm lunch you finish up eating at 9.00 pm in the evening which for most families is also too late.

I also combined my modified 18/6 plan with another plan by the name of **Alternative Day Fasting (ADF)** where I had breakfast every single day (so that I could take my medications), fast one day (breakfast - breakfast) and then ate three normal meals on the eating day. Then repeat the sequences again.

Another popular **Intermittent Fasting Plan** is the 5/2 plan which involves choosing any two 24 hour periods in each week as fasting periods and 5 days of eating. I have found the problem with this plan is it is too easy to put off the fasting days. Something comes up in your family life and you start to postpone the fast days and suddenly you haven't achieved the 2 days fasting in 7 days. With the 18/6 plan you will also be fasting 126 hours a week whereas with the 5/2 plan it is just 48 hours.

The following schedule is therefore based on my modified 18/6 plan but would also apply if you decide to follow the standard 16/8 plan. My suggestion is to set out an initial plan for the next 90 days which will divide up into three or five steps:

1. 7 days initial preparation

2. 30 days 18/6 plan (or the 16/8 plan)

3. 15 days of a 24/24 plan (alternate) or 15 days 18/6 plan (or the 16/8 plan)

4. 30 days 18/6 plan (or the 16/8 plan)

5. 7 days transition

Step 1

The first 7 days will be spent preparing yourself to begin the **Intermittent Fasting Plan**. During this time there are two main goals. Firstly, you will set regular times when you will be consuming your three meals - breakfast, lunch and dinner. My recommendation is breakfast at 7.00 am, lunch at 1.00 pm and dinner at 7.00 pm, but it could also be 6.00 am breakfast, lunch at 12.00 pm and dinner at 6.00 pm. It is important that these meals be eaten at the **same time each day**.

Secondly, you will start to reduce your intake of sugar and other carbohydrates (carbs) dramatically. In Appendix B you will find a list of things you should avoid consuming in Step 1 and throughout the whole plan to help you reduce your dependence on sugar. In Appendix A you will find a list of foods you can eat during these first 7 days as well as some simple suggestions for meals that are easy to prepare.

The important thing is to always be aware of this requirement. When you are out buying groceries **do not** be tempted to go for the foods which are labeled as "low fat" as they often contain sugars and other ingredients which are designed to provide more flavor. From this list in Appendix A you will be able to recognize the relationship between fat and low carbs. Unfortunately, we have been falsely educated that fat is bad for us. Sugars are bad, not fat.

Step 2

On day 8 you will begin with the actual **Intermittent Fasting Plan.** On this day you will eliminate either breakfast or dinner from the meals you consume. This can be a choice based upon a number of circumstances, the major one being your family or partner, whichever fits your particular social schedule. If dinner is the main time the family gets together at the meal table, then you would eliminate breakfast.

Vice-versa if breakfast is that meal then eliminate dinner. Lunch you will always be eating.

At this point you will be entering the phase where you will be eating in a 6-hour window (your eating period) and fasting for 18 hours (your fasting period). Based on how successful you have been implementing Step 1 will determine some of the effects you might feel during the first few days of Step 2. Some people complain about slight headaches, almost all about hunger and some about a lightheadedness. These should all subside after 3 or 4 days. We have included a couple of tips on how to deal with eventual hunger pangs. These will definitely disappear before the end of your first fasting week.

It is also of utmost importance that during the fasting period **only fluids** are consumed. Even a small trace of milk or cream in your coffee will destroy the fasting period. Sorry! In the Appendix there are suggestions for your meals during the eating period. The basis of these suggestions are low-carb ingredients and if you are familiar with this diet, then you can prepare your own alternatives.

After this first week of Step 2, you will start to see and feel the benefits of your plan. Most participants notice an increase in energy as the ketosis process kicks in (see page 34) and an improved mental awareness will be experienced. As you progress further into Step 2, you will be aware that hunger is no longer an issue. In fact it should disappear completely. You will look forward to your meals not because you are hungry but just because you will enjoy the eating experience.

To measure your progress regarding weight loss, **DO NOT STEP ON A SCALE**. Preferably take a piece of clothing (pants or a dress) that was a tight fit before you started and maybe have been the reason you started the program! After the second week in Step 2 you will begin to feel the difference which will give you extra motivation to keep going and focus on your goals.

Some people, including myself, found it interesting to observe how and where the fat elimination process takes place on your body. Standing in front of the mirror naked (not every day!) will allow you to watch this fascinating process. It will be different for all body types.

Step 3 (as an alternative)

At this point you will be 4 weeks into your **Intermittent Fasting Plan**. If you feel comfortable and are beginning to see results then there is no reason to change and just continue with Step 2 for another 45 days. If you feel like taking it up a notch and trying a different pattern of eating and fasting then I would recommend what I call the 24/24 plan or ADF (Alternate Day Fasting). This involves 24 hours of eating and 24 hours of fasting but with a twist. In the 24/24 plan you will be eating a breakfast (or dinner) in your fasting period and all three meals in your eating period.

Let's take an example. On Monday (your eating period) you will eat breakfast, lunch and dinner, keeping to your low-carb plan. On Tuesday (your fasting period) you will eat just breakfast. This means that your next meal will not be until breakfast on Wednesday, 24 hours of fasting later. Then on Wednesday again your three meals and then just breakfast on Thursday and so on. The reason this plan is a little more aggressive than the 18/6 plan is because your continuous fasting period is extended from 18 to 24 hours, allowing the ketosis effect more time to work.

If this 24/24 plan works for you then let it continue for as long as you wish. I would recommend at least coming back to the 18/6 plan two weeks before Step 5 begins.

Step 4

Depending on your decision about Step 3, Step 4 is just a continuation of Step 2.

Step 5

If you have really stuck to your plan, by this time you should be able to see and feel the difference. Depending on your starting point and where you were with your health (overweight, obese, flabby) this might be a good time to evaluate your progress. One thing you will definitely notice is, apart from no longer feeling hungry, your relationship to food will have changed. You will probably have lost the desire for something sweet and will have no trouble refusing an invitation to eat cakes and other calorie bombs. You will turn to fruits for that sweet taste.

In fact, by this time you will no longer want to eat because you are hungry but because you are looking forward to the social event eating can be and enjoying foods that are not loaded with masses of sugar. You will be saying no to pastas and potatoes and yes to more veggies. Personally, I have found that the hunger gremlin doesn't come back to haunt me, even though I am no longer actually fasting. If I do happen to overeat one day, I will include a 18/6 day the next day, no problem.

Again, if you feel totally at ease with your plan at this point there is no reason why you shouldn't continue. If you want to take a break then go back to your low-carb, three meals per day plan you started with in

Step 1. Having successfully completed your plan and achieved your goals, you will have acquired the confidence to do it all over again at any moment. This is one of the big advantages of the **Intermittent Fasting Plan**. You never have to go back to where you were before. I don't know anyone who has eliminated all of the benefits of fasting and put the weight back on again.

Please remember, the things you learned about yourself and food are important. Even if you decide to break your fast for a while and go back to "normal" life again, continue with a low-sugar, low-carb nutrition program. If you feel for it, throw in a day or two of fasting each month. It will help you maintain the gains you have achieved.

7. FASTING TIPS

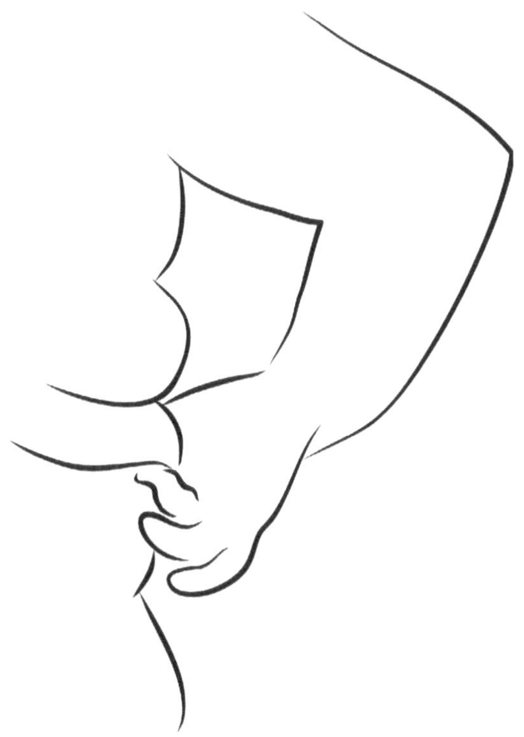

Fear Of Hunger

One of the biggest fears people have when considering any fasting program is the fear of hunger. It's the one thing that might even prevent you from starting. This fear is real, so is the hunger. However, I am here to tell you, it **will** subside and finally disappear (in my case never to return). As I mentioned at the start of the fasting plan, it is important you follow the suggestions outlined in Step 1, the first week before the actual fast. The goal of this first week is to burn off as much glucose (sugar) in your system as possible before Step 2. This will enable the ketosis process to kick in with full force at the beginning of your fast and will enable you to benefit from all the advantages of new energy and mental focus that ketosis brings.

There are a few tricks one can use to minimize the effects of hunger during the first week of Step 2. Drink as much fluids as possible. Always have a bottle of water at hand. Coffee and tea without any additives (sugar or milk) is helpful and one trick is to add one teaspoon of coconut oil to the tea or coffee. It gives it a sweeter flavor which tricks the brain and your stomach into believing you have ingested something. This then reduces the hunger hormone signaling from your stomach. The coconut oil is pure fat and will not interrupt your fasting period. Milk and cream, no matter how little, contain small amounts of carbs and will spike an insulin response and interrupt the ketosis process.

Another trick is to brush your teeth. Apart from being a good idea anyway, brushing your teeth puts a fresh taste in your mouth and will have the same effect as the coconut oil. The same would apply if you can find sugar-free, carb-free chewing gum…as long as you don't swallow it! One thing you might notice is you could experience a spell of "bad breath" during the fast. This is caused by the body eliminating the byproducts of fat burning through your breath and is a good sign your body is in its state of ketosis. Typically, this problem disappears after a couple of weeks.

The other thing to remember is that of the 18 hours fasting period you will be sleeping between 6 and 8 hours and will still be burning fat. In the majority of cases the hunger problem will subside and disappear after the third day, with women sometimes a little longer. Then it will be plain sailing and you will be asking yourself "why haven't I tried this fasting thing before?".

A final trick is to overcome the hunger that could occur in the evening is just plan to go to bed a little earlier. You will probably start to feel a little more tired during the first few days and welcome the chance to hit the sack a little earlier.

And finally an observation I experienced after my first fast was over. We have all been horrified by the terrible pictures we have all seen on the TV and in the media of starving people and children in places like Africa. They have often been without food for weeks or months at a time. The emotion these pictures ignite within us is how terrible it must be suffer from a constant hunger. I now realize these poor individuals are not suffering from hunger but from devastating malnutrition. Their hunger hormones no longer exist. Not a pretty thought but it just goes to show how superficial our western way of life has become. It also reminds us that, in our attempt to lose weight, we should perhaps contribute some small amount to those people in the world that need to gain weight.

Exercise

Exercise is not something I address at length in this book as it is a very broad subject and can range from pure athletics to weight training or just going for a walk. What I do recommend is at least 3 - 4 days of very moderate exercise. This could include walking briskly for 30 minutes on each of the 3 - 4 days as a minimum. For those who are used to a more rigorous routine, there is no reason to stop. In the first week of fasting you might experience a feeling of extreme tiredness as your body transitions and adjusts from burning glucose for energy to burning fat (ketosis).

In fact, the more exercise you perform, the quicker and more effective the ketosis process becomes. Many top athletes have discovered that getting their bodies into a mode of ketosis improves their performance dramatically as their bodies prefer this source of energy over glucose. For those who train with weights and/or want to build muscle at the same time as burning fat, experts recommend doing this about an hour before a meal. Personally, I recommend for non-body builders, get started with your fasting plan first, remove some of the fat and then slowly work into some light weight training, 20 to 30 days into the plan. This you can do at home with some inexpensive dumbbells. Riding your bike is also a great exercise in combination with the light weight training. It helps build leg muscle.

Buying Groceries

One of the keys to eating the right products and preparing the right meals starts already in the supermarket. There are thousands of websites which give tons of good advice on healthy products and their nutritional values so I am going to limit my comments here to general good practices. The first rule in healthy eating according to **"Intermittent Fasting Best Practices"** is to <u>avoid processed food</u> at all costs as much as possible. When entering the store or supermarket, head straight for the fresh foods department. At best the bio foods section.

You will notice that fresh meat, fish, fruits and vegetables do not carry any nutritional labelling. They are not required to. Of course, there are always things that can be purchased as packaged food and can still be healthy. However, it is important you become familiar with and know how to read the nutritional information these processed foods must carry. After all, they have originated from a factory production line and are not fresh off the farm.

We have already addressed the question of sugar enough and it is aways the first thing I look for when I read the nutritional labels. In fact I have developed a real hatred for foods that contain more than 5g. of sugar on 100g. (5%). Again, there is loads of information on how to read these labels on the Internet and, even if you were not used to paying attention to this before, it won't take long before you get the hang of it and become an expert. Carbs, fats, proteins and sugar.

One resistance I often hear from people on smaller incomes is living on "bio" foods is much more expensive. This is true, although with the popularity of healthy eating on the increase, it has created more competition and all of the major supermarket chains now have a growing "bio" section. My reply to this objection is, when you are into your fast, you will be eating less and therefore able to survive on a reduced budget. What you save on the quantity you can invest in the quality of what you feed your body. Better for you and your family.

Finally, with the growing interest in bio foods I have noticed more and more farmers and small local businesses getting in on the act. The popularity of local markets is on the increase. I no longer buy my eggs from a supermarket but from a local guy with his own chickens! Even meats and fish I select either from the local market or over the counter and no longer from the prepackaged shelves. This often helps support the local farmers and not farmers somewhere in South America!

Eating Out

For those of us who cannot always eat at home, one might think eating out could pose a problem and even a threat to our fasting program. This does not have to be the case. All it requires is a little discipline.

In its simplest form, all you have to do is memorize the list of things listed in Appendix A. Slip a copy in your pocket if that is easier. Most restaurants are familiar with clients on all sorts of diets and are happy to adjust the dishes to fit your requirements. Of course, if you decide to visit an establishment which only serves pizzas, this could be a problem.

If you finish up in a food court, then avoid the pizzas, pastas, burgers and the like. Better alternatives are the Asian cuisines. If possible, replace the rice with more vegetables and if that is not possible, don't eat all the rice! If you are really stuck at McDonalds, then order their chicken nuggets and/or one of their salad bowls. Even McDonalds is trying to cater to the growing health conscious segment!

8. AND NOW...

Maintenance Program

And now that you have completed your fast and have reached your goals, there is a time thereafter! You have shed off that extra fat to the point you are now happy with your own body, you are more confident, with more energy and a desire to get more out of life. This is not a lot of BS but how you will actually feel now that you have completed the plan and have your eating under control.

It is time to focus on how to maintain your new health and make sure you don't fall back into old habits. In my case it has not been difficult. During the 90 days of my first **Intermittent Fasting Plan** I not only changed my eating times, I also changed my eating habits. I learned how dangerous too much sugar is to my health and now avoid it as much as I can. I learned how to read the food labels and now buy my groceries accordingly. I avoid buying processed food as much as I can and invested in a smoothie mixer which I now use to prepare delicious, healthy nutrition.

As I have said before, **Intermittent Fasting** is not just a method to burn fat fast and get healthier, it is just as much a change in lifestyle. I have always been very active but now I build my bike rides and evening walks into my schedule. The amazing increase I experience in my mental focus has meant I read (and write) a lot more. It is hard to describe but I just have the feeling of being more than 10 years younger!

Getting back to the fast itself, my advice is not to exaggerate with the length of your fast no matter how much weight you might want to lose. The danger is the success you will experience will encourage you to keep going, meaning you just keep fasting without a time limit.

In my own case, I had set my goals for my first fast and wanted to achieve them within 90 days. This happened quickly and because I found **Intermittent Fasting** to be actually very easy, I was tempted to adjust my goals and just keep going. I felt great with lots of energy and an incredible mental focus. But something told me to ease of a little and transition into what I would call a **maintenance program**.

What I recommend to everyone, is return to the low-carb diet which I promote for the preparation phase in Week 1. If you are looking for an plan with ideas and recipes on what to eat then do a search on the web for a **ketogenic diet**. There are lots of them out there and they limit the sugar and balance the proteins your body needs.

Another suggestion to consider is to increase your exercise program somewhat. In my case, I invested a few dollars in some dumbbells (at home) so I can start to build more muscles now that I can see them better! For your health, it is not necessary to go crazy with health club subscriptions and workout programs even though you will come across bodybuilders who promote **Intermittent Fasting** to build those ripped bodies. They may look great but they require high maintenance!

Your Powerful Weapon

Another positive result of completing your first **Intermittent Fasting Plan** is you now have a powerful tool at your fingertips to stay healthy and slim for the rest of your life. A natural reaction to finishing the plan is to indulge occasionally in some of the "pleasures of life" again. This could include feasting yourself full at certain festivals such as Thanksgiving or celebrating birthdays with a few extra glasses of stronger liquid refreshment. It might include vacations eating out in exotic restaurants or an occasional ice sundae on the beach.

It doesn't matter. Now you can quickly "recover" by fitting in a day or two of **Intermittent Fasting** into your normal schedule again and undo the "damage".

Many intermittent fasters just include some form of fast into their weekly schedule on a permanent basis. Some of my friends have just eliminated breakfast completely from their schedule which means they have a daily 16/8 or 18/6 **Intermittent Fast** depending on when they eat lunch and dinner.

Personally, breakfast with my wife on the balcony overlooking an incredible lakeside view is a highlight of every day so we prefer just skip dinner occasionally. We have also found by skipping dinner our bodies stay in a more rested state in the evening which promotes a better night's sleep.

For those who are drastically overweight and are utilizing **Intermittent Fasting** to lose large amounts of fat, it is probably advisable to break down the goals into a number of different stages, preferably under medical supervision. 90-day fasting periods seems to be the number many are sticking to and in my experience it is neither too short nor too long. With one week preparation and one week transition this means it is just 10 weeks of actual fasting.

A break of 4 weeks between each fasting period provides enough time to analyze the results. If you are super serious about your health then visit your doctor to do an "annual checkup" before you begin your fast and get your blood markers recorded so you can follow your progress.

Conclusion

Now is the time to take action. I hope I have provided you enough information to convince you to give **Intermittent Fasting** a try. It costs you nothing, is easy to do and the results are incredible. All it takes is a decision. A decision to burn fat, lose weight and live a more fulfilling, healthier and longer life. You owe it to yourself and to your body - this wonderful machine which provides you with the life you are living. It will respond and pay you back ten times over! As you experience the results, make sure to pass on this information to the people you care about and be part of this revolution to change the world of health. **Here's to your success!**

9. APPENDICES

Appendix A - Things To Avoid Eating

Appendix B - Things To Plan Eating

Appendix C - Meal Ideas

Appendix D - Scientific References

Appendix E - Video Links

Appendix F - Biohacking & Nutrigenomics

Appendix A - Things To Avoid Eating

Let's address first the things you should **absolutely avoid at all costs** right from the beginning. This is the list you should avoid in Step 1 of your plan and preferably during the complete plan. These are things we often consume and which include masses of carbs and sugar:

- all types of pastas and rice (sorry!)

- all varieties of potatoes

- all white breads

- all cakes, flans, pies, desserts (you get the picture)

- no pizzas (sorry!)

- all types of fruit not on the list

- all alcoholic beverages, no wine, no beer

- cream and/or sugar in your coffee/tea

- all fruit juices and sodas

- types of vegetables not on the list of Appendix B

- all salad dressings (only olive oil and vinegar allowed)

The sooner you depart from the past, and in particular from the habit of eating these foods, the faster you will reach the point beyond hunger. This makes **Intermittent Fasting** not only more pleasurable, it makes it also more effective

Appendix B - Things To Plan Eating

Here is a list of meats that can form the basis of your meals both during the Step 1, the preparation phase, as well the meals you consume during your fast:

Source of Proteins			
	Fats (g)	Carbs (g)	Protein (g)
Ground Beef	23	0	20
Ribeye Steak	25	0	27
Bacon	51	0	13
Pork Chop	18	0	30
Chicken Thigh	20	0	17
Chicken Breast	1	0	26
Salmon	15	0	23
Ground Lamb	27	0	19
Liver	5	0	19
Eggs	5	0.5	6

Here is a list of the types of vegetables/fruits that you can use to accompany the meats as part of the meal:

Recommended Fruits and Vegetables			
	Fats (g)	Carbs (g)	Protein (g)
Cabbage	0	6	2
Cauliflower	0	6	5
Broccoli	1	7	5
Spinach	0	1	3
Lettuce	1	2	2
Green Bell Pepper	0	5	1
Mushrooms	0	4	6
Green Beans	0	4	2
Blackberries	1	8	2
Raspberries	1	8	2

After the main course, get creative with some of these ingredients to prepare a dessert or a cheese board:

Recommended Dairy Products			
	Fats (g)	Carbs (g)	Protein (g)
Heavy Cream	12	0	0
Greek Yoghurt	1	1	3
Mayonnaise	20	0	0
Cottage Cheese	1	1	4
Cream Cheese	9	1	2
Mascarpone	13	0	2
Brie	8	0	6
Aged Cheddar	9	0	7
Parmesan	7	1	10
Mozzarella	5	1	5

Or if you <u>must</u> bake a cake...don't go too wild and don't forget, during the fast **ONLY** eat these during your eating period!

Various Flours For Baking Cakes			
	Fats (g)	Carbs (g)	Protein (g)
Almond Flour	12	0	0
Coconut Flour	1	1	3
Chia Seed Meal	20	0	0
Flaxseed Meal	1	1	4

Finally, use these nuts if you really must snack during meals **BUT** only during Step 1. There is **NO SNACKING** during the fast.

Choice of Nuts			
	Fats (g)	Carbs (g)	Protein (g)
Macadamia Nuts	43	3	4
Brazil Nuts	37	3	8
Pecans	41	3	5
Almonds	28	5	12
Hazelnut	36	3	9

Appendix C - Meal Ideas

By applying some of the ingredients mentioned in Appendix B, as well as my own personal experience during my fast, I would like to share a couple of simple solutions to meals you can eat and/or prepare during the eating periods of your **Intermittent Fast**. If you keep to the plan, one thing you will definitely experience is your relationship to food will change. Before fasting, your decisions to eat are determined by routines and hunger. After you get past the "hunger stage" of fasting (on average about three days into the fast) you will only eat because you want to, or because you have planned a meal, not because you have to (hunger).

What has a "good" breakfast in the past looked like? For me it was a bowl of cereal (laden with sugar), an orange juice (loaded with even more sugar), followed by some bread and marmalade or something else sweet. All sugar bombs! This is an example of where the food industry has carried out a very successful campaign. "Breakfast is the most important meal of the day" was the motto. They then loaded the supermarket shelves with sweetened foods to boost their profits and damage our health.

So what are the alternatives? Once you start your fast and decide to eliminate breakfast, this will no longer be a problem. If you keep breakfast as one of your two meals then this is what I would recommend. We are used to eating eggs for breakfast. Replace your one boiled egg with more eggs. A simple solution that looks like a real meal is scrambled eggs on toast.

Crack three or four eggs into a bowl, add a small amount of salt, lots of pepper and a splash of full-fat milk and whisk it with a fork (or mixer!). Warm up your frying pan on a medium heat and melt some real butter. Slice up a few of tomatoes (based on their size) and fry them in the pan for a minute or two. Pour over the egg mix, turn off the heat and then stir the mixture around until it is ready. Make sure it doesn't get too dry. Prepare your toast and you have a breakfast that not only looks delicious, smells good, it is very tasty and satisfying. Drink your cup of coffee without sugar or milk and you will be set for the morning.

For those of you who still love the idea of a cereal bowl (including me!), this is what I did and still do. Buy rolled grain with 4 - 5 grain types included. Shake your portion into a cereal bowl, sprinkle the following ingredients over it: finely chopped coconut, a few sultanas, finely chopped walnuts and grated linseed or quinoa. Mix everything together and pour over your full-fat milk and let it sit five minutes. It will be the healthiest "musli" you have ever tried, almost no sugar and very satisfying.

Another alternative for breakfast which I use is crispbread with cheese. Light and satisfying. Also something one can prepare quickly and eat on the way to work, with coffee-to-go. But during a fast, many people find the best meal to eliminate in the 18/6 plan is breakfast. In the morning we have other things on our minds such as getting ready for work or driving the kids to school. Time will fly anyway, especially if your next planned meal is already at 12.00 pm!

Looking forward to lunch, it is in almost all fasting plans the one meal you will always be eating. It is therefore as equally important from a fasting and a nutrition standpoint. The basis can be almost any of the meats or fish. They can be grilled or fried. If fried, then only in olive oil, real butter or coconut oil. Then you can add any of the vegetables on the list in any quantities you desire. To fill up the plate add more vegetables! A green salad on the side for vitamins but only with a dressing of oil and vinegar.

Then we arrive at dinner. Depending on the fasting plan you choose this might be your main meal of the day, maybe with the whole family. Just bear in mind not to eat much later than 7.00 pm to make sure you maximize on your fasting period and not to have to adjust your next meal (lunch) to much later than 1.00 pm.

For those of us who are not gourmet cooks, keep things simple. Scrambled eggs on toast and the bowl of cereal (as shown above!) can be consumed anytime not just for breakfast. One way to create tremendous nutritional value with the minimum of work is to start preparing smoothies. My investment in a smoothie blender was probably (after fasting) the best thing I could have done for my body. Now I am able to prepare a liquid meal which is a nutritional "bomb" by throwing in fruits and vegetables into my blender and pressing the button. Delicious and refreshing!

For those who like be in the kitchen and cook gourmet meals, either for lunch or dinner, then a good resource for recipes would be to google "ketogenic recipes". There you will find thousands of suggestions for recipes that fulfill the ketogenic requirements for a low-carb diet, most of them using the ingredients mentioned in Appendix B. Some people completely integrate the ketogenic diet with **Intermittent Fasting** for maximum results.

Many of us tend not to eat a full-blown meal at dinnertime and take more of a snack. In this case a great solution is to load up a platter with various cheeses, meats and fish for a good-looking and delicious presentation with minimal work. Consume these delicacies with various types of crispbread and for decoration use olives, tomatoes, celery and/or radishes.

Appendix D - Scientific References

Nobel Prize For Medicine 2016:

http://bit.ly/2NL6m4y

Fasting: Molecular Mechanisms and Clinical Applications:

http://bit.ly/2uhlBZY

Fasting Cycles Retard Growth of Tumors and Sensitize a Range of Cancer Cell Types to Chemotherapy:

http://bit.ly/2ubneJv

Intermittent Fasting and Obesity:

http://bit.ly/2m7OoMU

Short-term fasting induces profound neuronal autophagy:

http://bit.ly/2KWC7cl

Energy Intake and Exercise as Determinants of Brain Health and Vulnerability to Injury and Disease:

http://bit.ly/2KMY3r4

Protective effects of short-term dietary restriction in surgical stress and chemotherapy:

http://bit.ly/2KZolFP

Appendix E - Video Links

Eat, Fast And Live Longer - The BBC Documentary

https://vimeo.com/278329970

Introduction To Fasting (56 Minutes):

https://vimeo.com/254442742

Meet the woman who lost 50 pounds through Intermittent Fasting:

https://vimeo.com/265431243

The Process Of Ketosis:

https://vimeo.com/255008799

The Perfect Treatment For Type 2 Diabetes, Dr. Jason Fung:

https://vimeo.com/257190501

Appendix F - Biohacking & Nutrigenomics

Biohacking is a terminology which has only recently emerged. It relates to a new branch of biological science by the name of Nutrigenomics. This involves the study of how gene expression can be manipulated by the things we ingest (and also don't ingest). In many cases genes can also be impacted by stress in the form of physical exercise.

This trend is a relatively recent phenomenon and has only emerged and been made possible as a result of the development of new technology which allows scientists to study the human body at a micro-cellular level. This has brought into question many of the old theories scientists had been assuming for decades. Such theories had evolved as a result of researchers making certain assumptions without having access to these new technologies to be able to validate them.

Now many of the mysteries of the human body are starting to be explained and understood like never before. One important discovery is we are able to manipulate our gene expression with the things we eat. Scientists are gradually getting answers to how things go wrong in our bodies, leading to poor health, disease and death. This is leading to non-pharmaceutical solutions to illness and a new approach to preventing and curing rather than treating diseases.

I remember reading many years ago that for every disease and ailment mankind suffers from there is a cure somewhere on the planet. For centuries man has been trying to cure diseases with plants and herbs by trial and error and now it seems this may well be the best solution as modern science is on the path to prove many of their theories to be valid.

In this book on **Intermittent Fasting** I have been addressing what happens when we basically stop eating or reduce drastically the intake of sugar and carbohydrates. Our bodies react to what could be described as a "stress" state and adapts to the new situation, takes a timeout and sets a number of processes in motion to correct the mistakes of the past and adapt to the new situation. Scientists are now able to study and document what actually happens to our cellular structures in this situation. Suddenly, new knowledge emerges which rebukes some of the old doctrines we have lived by.

In the Science Chapter, I describe what happens in the process called autophagy. This is a very recent discovery. For centuries, scientists had no idea this process even took place. You stop eating, the body takes a break and uses the time to repair itself. Only this would be reason enough to start and frequently use an **Intermittent Fasting Plan**. This is better than eating ourselves to obesity. **Intermittent Fasting** can prevent the body from silently developing any number of deadly diseases without us finding out until it might be too late.

I have taken **Intermittent Fasting** to the next step and have developed a concept called **"The Biohack Formula"** which lays out the four components which make up the biohacking process. These four "Pillars" of the formula lay out the four things we should be paying attention to in order to live a long, healthy and disease-free life. **Intermittent Fasting** is just one of these four pillars:

1. **Nutrition** - feeding our body with the right nutrients

2. **Intermittent Fasting** - planning when we eat

3. **Regular exercise** - keeping in shape

4. **Triggers** - targeting planned responses

In this book I have focused on the subject of **Intermittent Fasting** because it helps us to correct some of the mistakes we have made in the past such as unhealthy nutrition. It is also a relatively new phenomenon which is not being promoted by any of the big industry players and is only spreading through word-of-mouth advertising.

However, each of these four subjects merits a book in its own right and in fact on the subjects of nutrition and exercise there is enough material available. I am writing a book on the subject of biohacking which will be coming out shortly and which will address all the pillars and in particular the one on **Triggers and Nutrigenomics**.

For more information and to register for my new book:

"The Biohacking Formula"

http://biohackformula.com